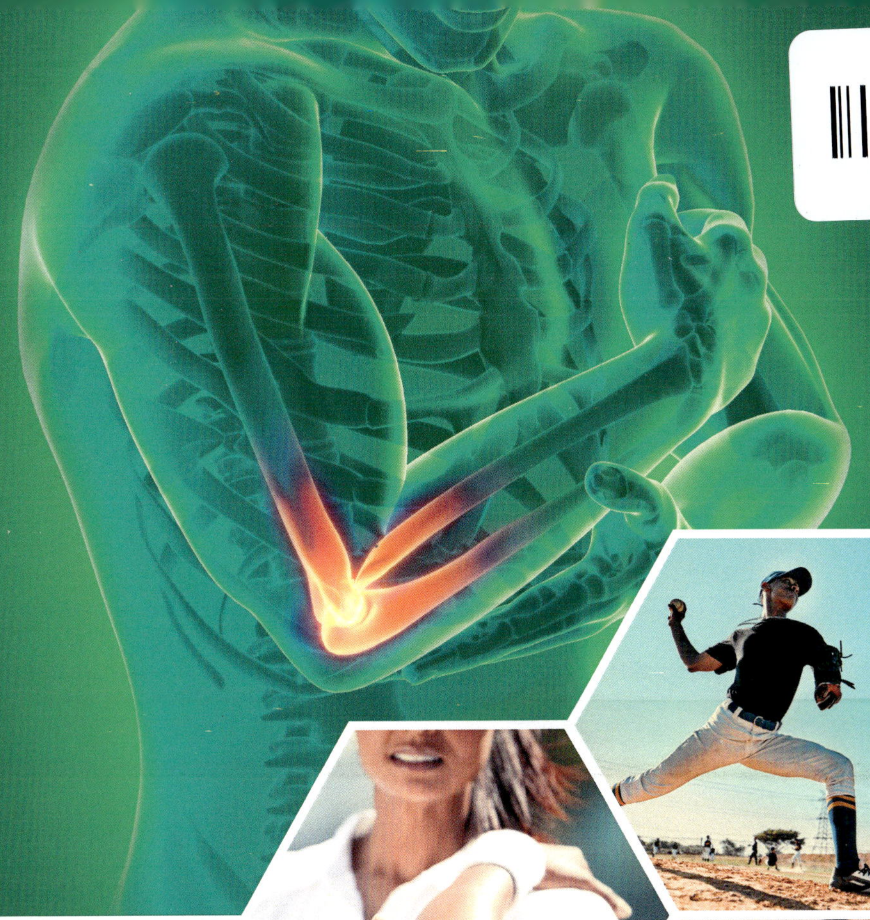

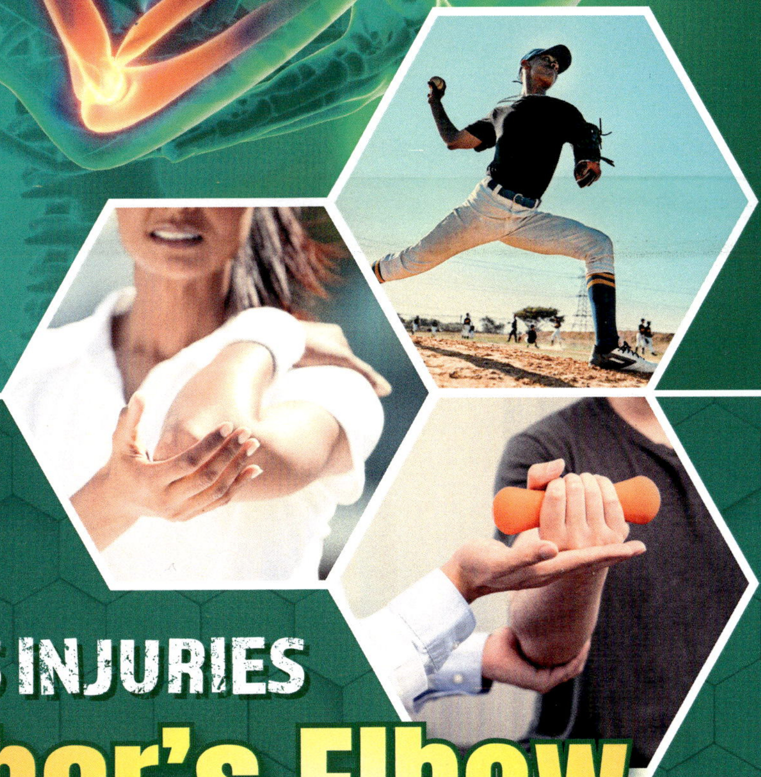

India James

SPORTS INJURIES

Pitcher's Elbow

A Crabtree Forest Book

Crabtree Publishing
crabtreebooks.com

School-to-Home Support for Caregivers and Teachers

This appealing book is designed to teach students about core subject areas. Students will build upon what they already know about the subject and engage in topics that they want to learn more about. Here are a few guiding questions to help readers build comprehension skills. Possible answers appear here in red.

Before Reading:

- What do I know about pitcher's elbow injuries?
  - *I know that many baseball players get pitcher's elbow*
  - *I know that many professional baseball players have surgery for pitcher's elbow*
- What do I want to learn about this topic?
  - *I want to know what muscles and bones are involved in pitcher's elbow injuries*
  - *I want to know how to prevent pitcher's elbow*

During Reading:

- I'm curious to know...
  - *I'm curious to know who can get pitcher's elbow*
  - *I'm curious to know how to recover from pitcher's elbow*
- How is this like something I already know?
  - *I know that pitcher's elbow happens from throwing*
  - I know that pitcher's elbow can be a severe (bad) injury

After Reading:

- What was the author trying to teach me?
  - *The author was trying to teach me what parts of my body are hurt by pitcher's elbow*
  - *The author was trying to teach me ways of treating pitcher's elbow*
- How did the photographs and captions help me understand more?
  - *The drawings of elbow bones, muscles, and tendons helped me understand the parts of my body involved with pitcher's elbow*
  - *The pictures of MRI,* ***X-ray,*** *and* ***ultrasound*** *machines helped me understand what tests a doctor might use to understand my pitcher's elbow*

Table of Contents

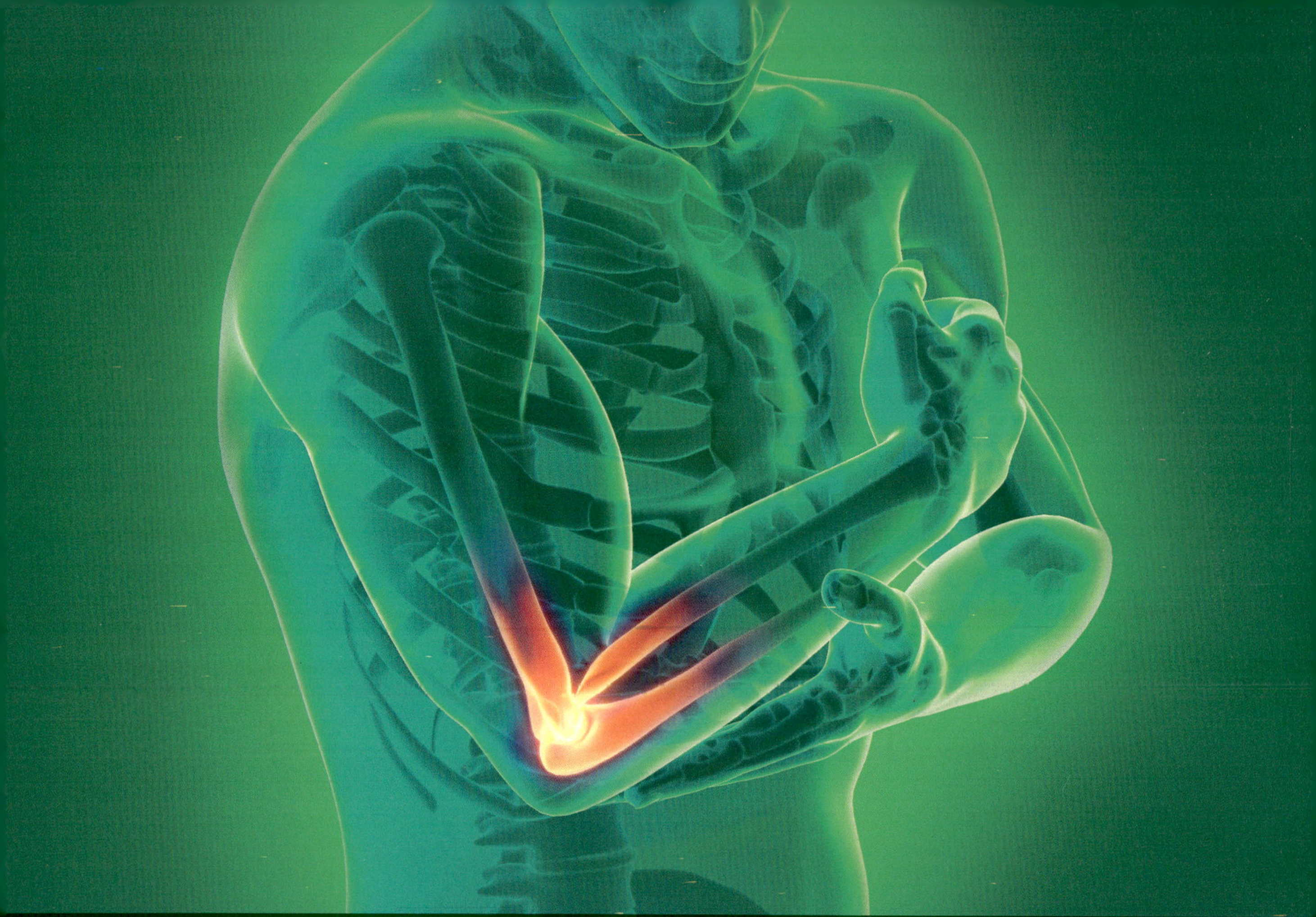

Chapter 1: What Is Pitcher's Elbow?

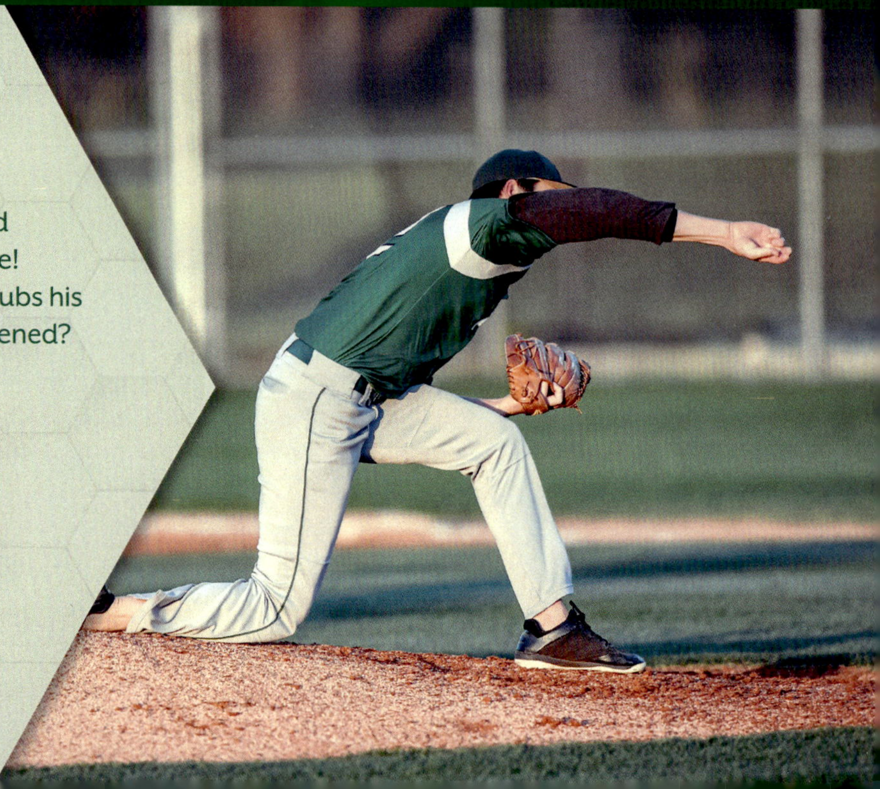

Out on the mound, the pitcher raises his leg. His arm winds back. His hand comes up, over his shoulder, and he flings the ball forward. It speeds past the batter and lands in the catcher's mitt. Strike three! But back on the mound, the pitcher rubs his elbow. He winces in pain. What happened?

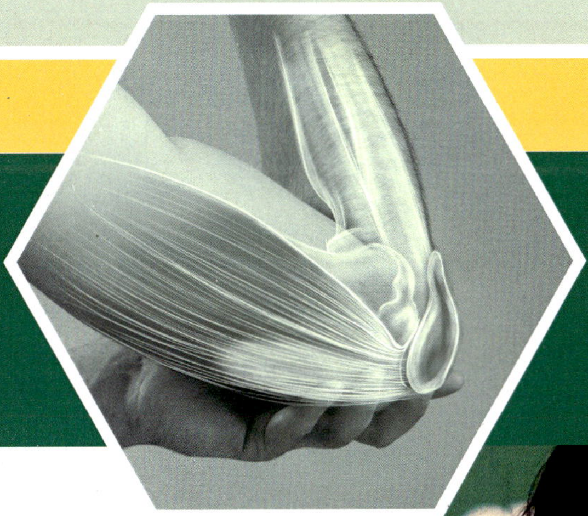

Pitcher's Elbow

This athlete is suffering from an elbow injury called pitcher's elbow. Sometimes it's also called a Tommy John injury. This injury happens when too much strain is put on the elbow too many times.

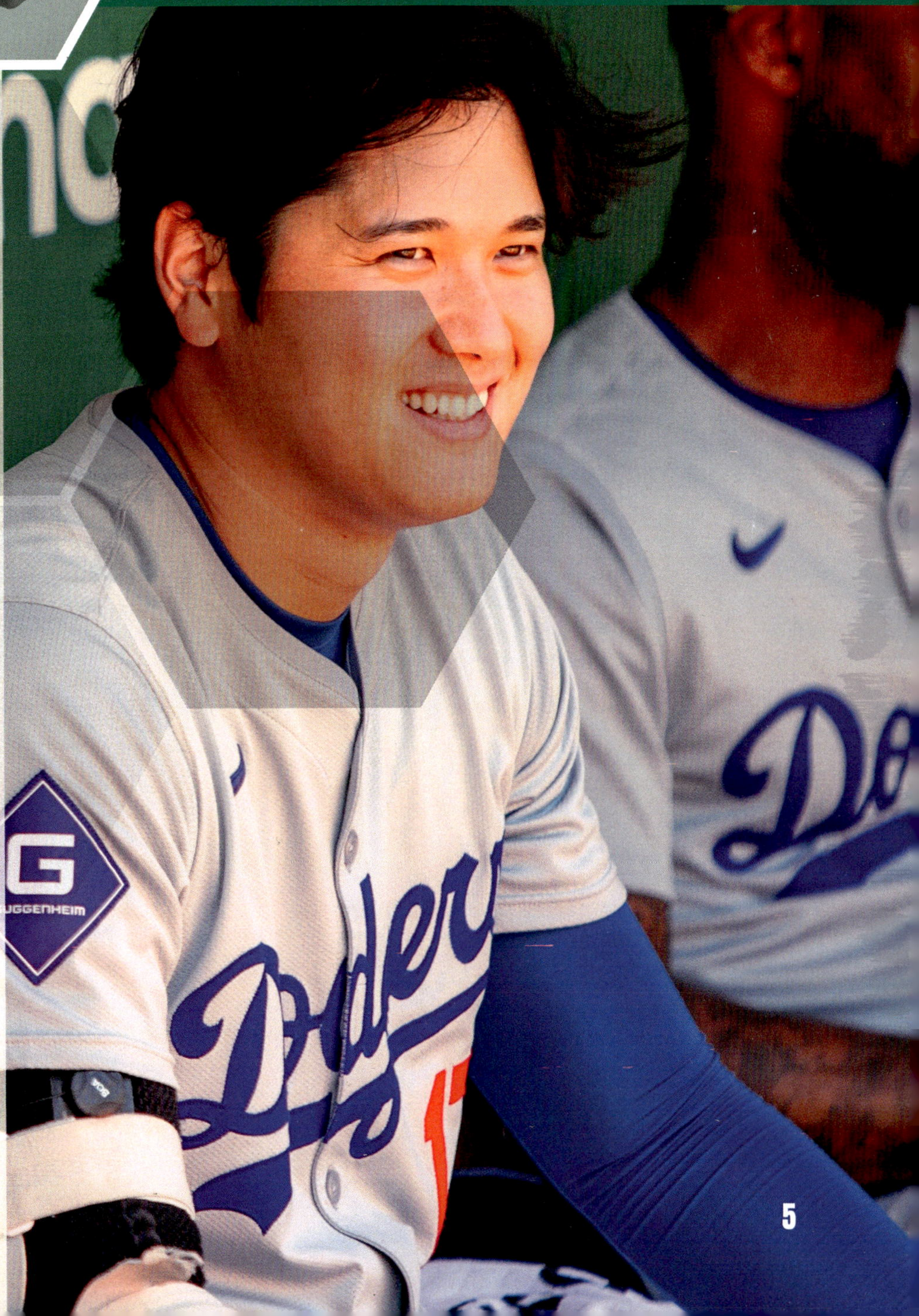

More than 1,000 professional baseball pitchers have had Tommy John surgery and returned to playing baseball, including Shohei Ohtani. The surgery was named after Major League Baseball (MLB) pitcher Tommy John, who was the first to have it in 1974.

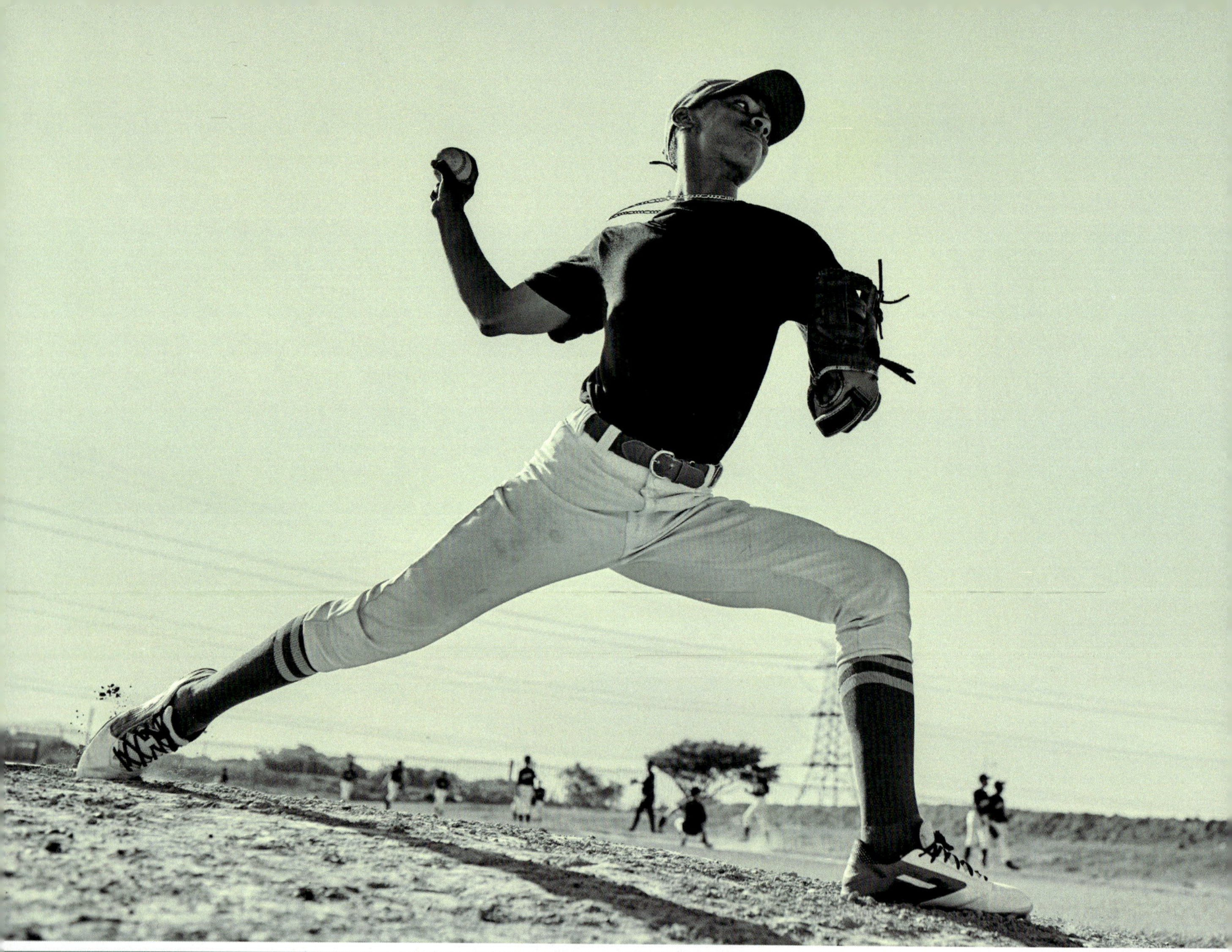

Pitcher's elbow is a common injury. It can happen to any athlete who plays a throwing sport, like quarterbacks in football or javelin throwers in track and field, but it is especially common in baseball. In just the first half of 2023, 31 major league pitchers had surgery to repair this injury. But you don't have to be professional athlete to get it. Even people playing sports just for fun can get a pitcher's elbow injury.

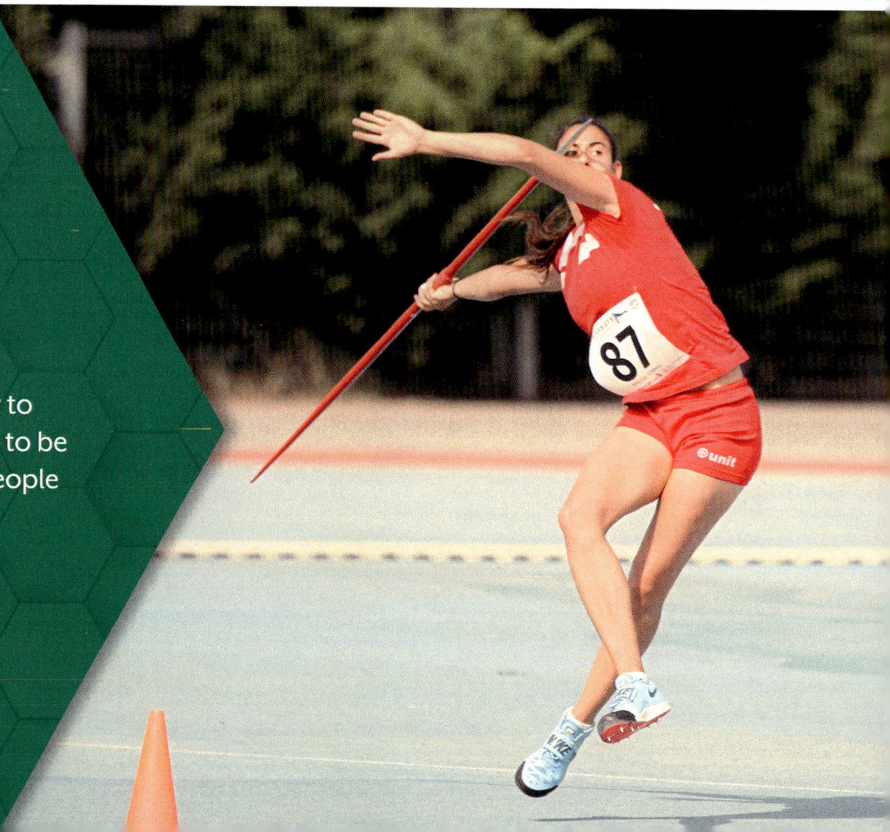

Doctors, athletic trainers, and other medical professionals understand how to help athletes when they have pitcher's elbow. They can help an athlete recover. You can help prevent pitcher's elbow by understanding what causes it.

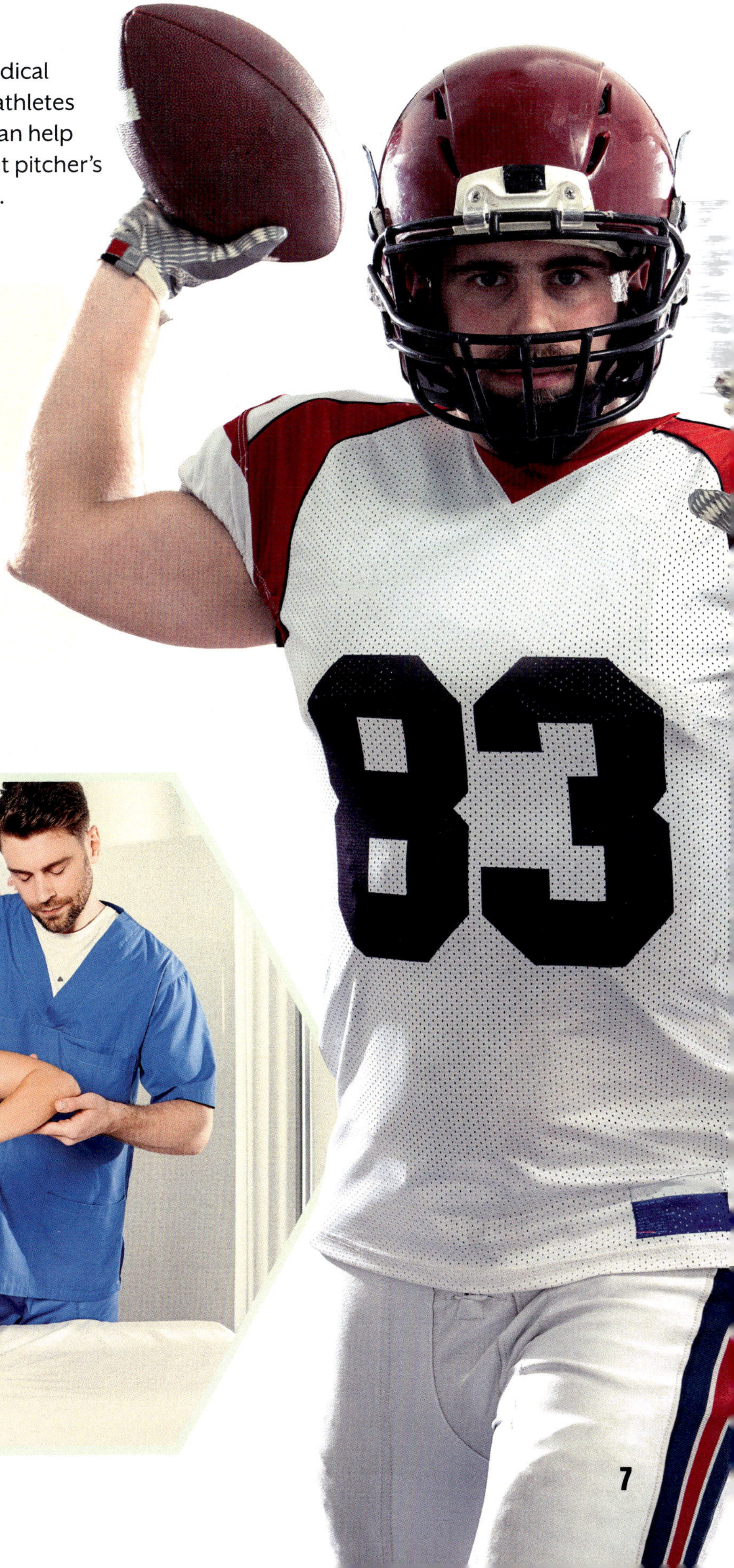

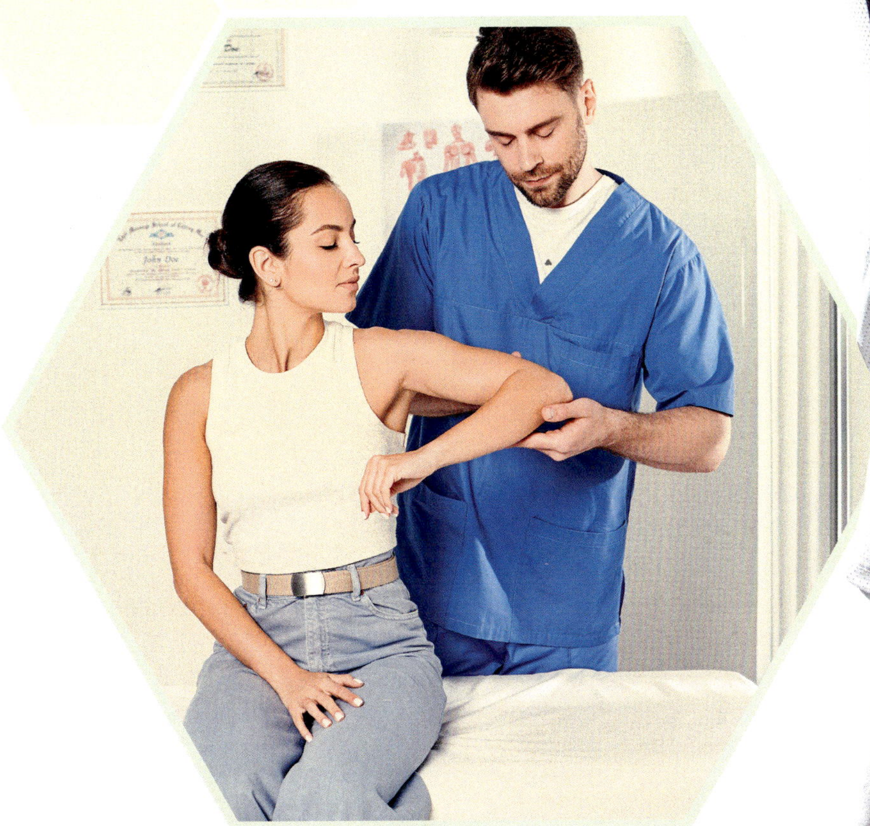

Chapter 2: Anatomy

Anatomy describes body parts and how they work together. Understanding how injuries happen starts with knowing the way muscles, bones, and **ligaments** function.

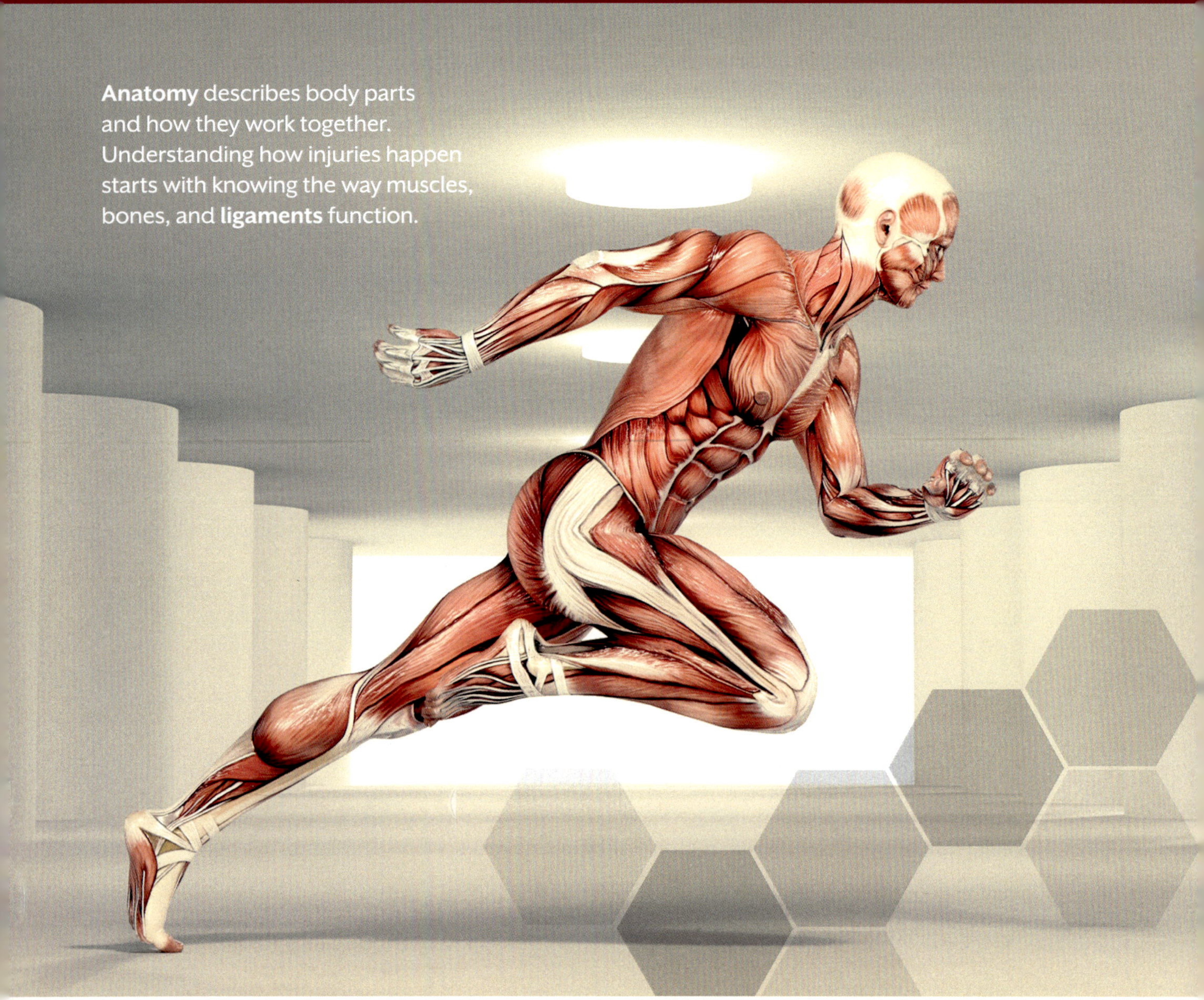

Bones

Hard **bones** support your body like a metal frame holds up a building. Some bones, such as your rib cage, also work to protect your soft organs.

Three bones are important to a pitcher's elbow injury

- **Humerus**
- **Radius**
- **Ulna**

The humerus is the long bone in your upper arm.

The radius is the thicker and shorter of the two forearm bones. The radius is on the thumb side of your forearm.

The ulna is the longer and thinner of the two forearm bones. The ulna is on the little finger, or pinky, side of your forearm.

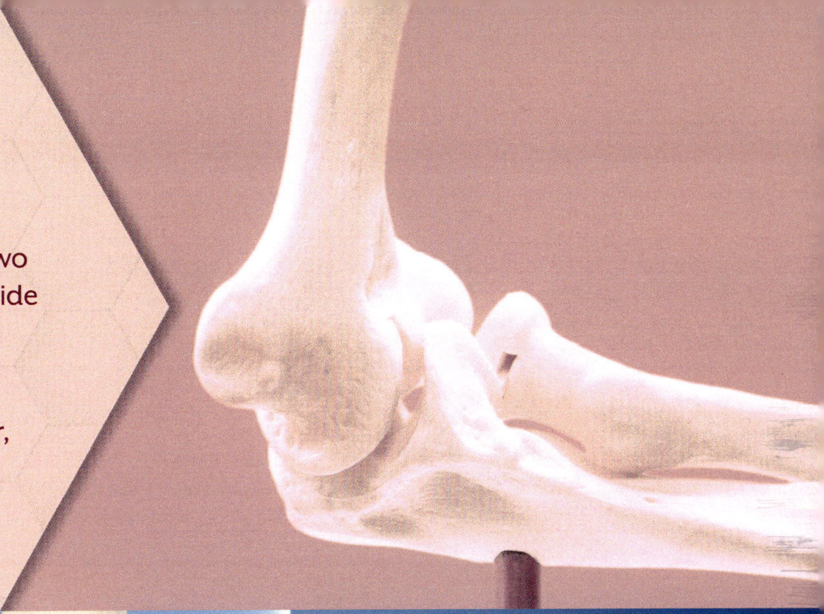

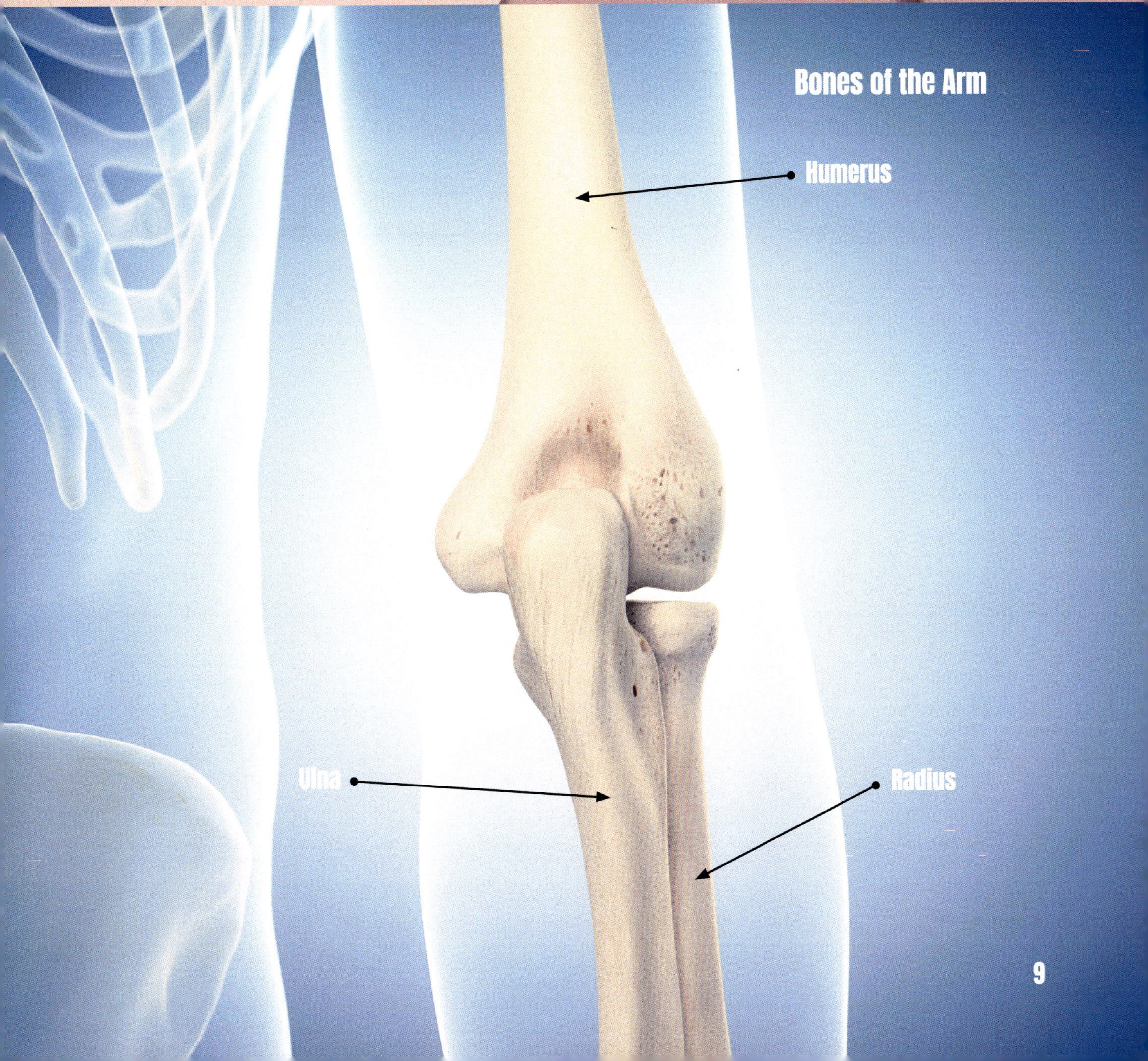

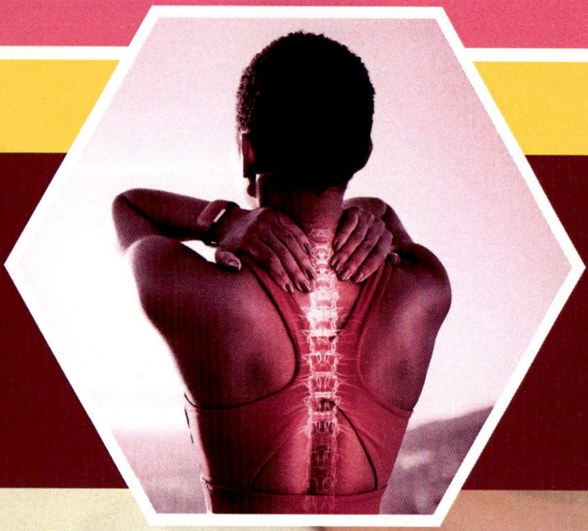

Joints

The place where two or more bones come together is called a joint. Some **joints,** such as the bones of your skull, don't move. Other joints, such as the bones of your spine, move just a little bit. However, many joints in your body move a lot. These are called **mobile joints**.

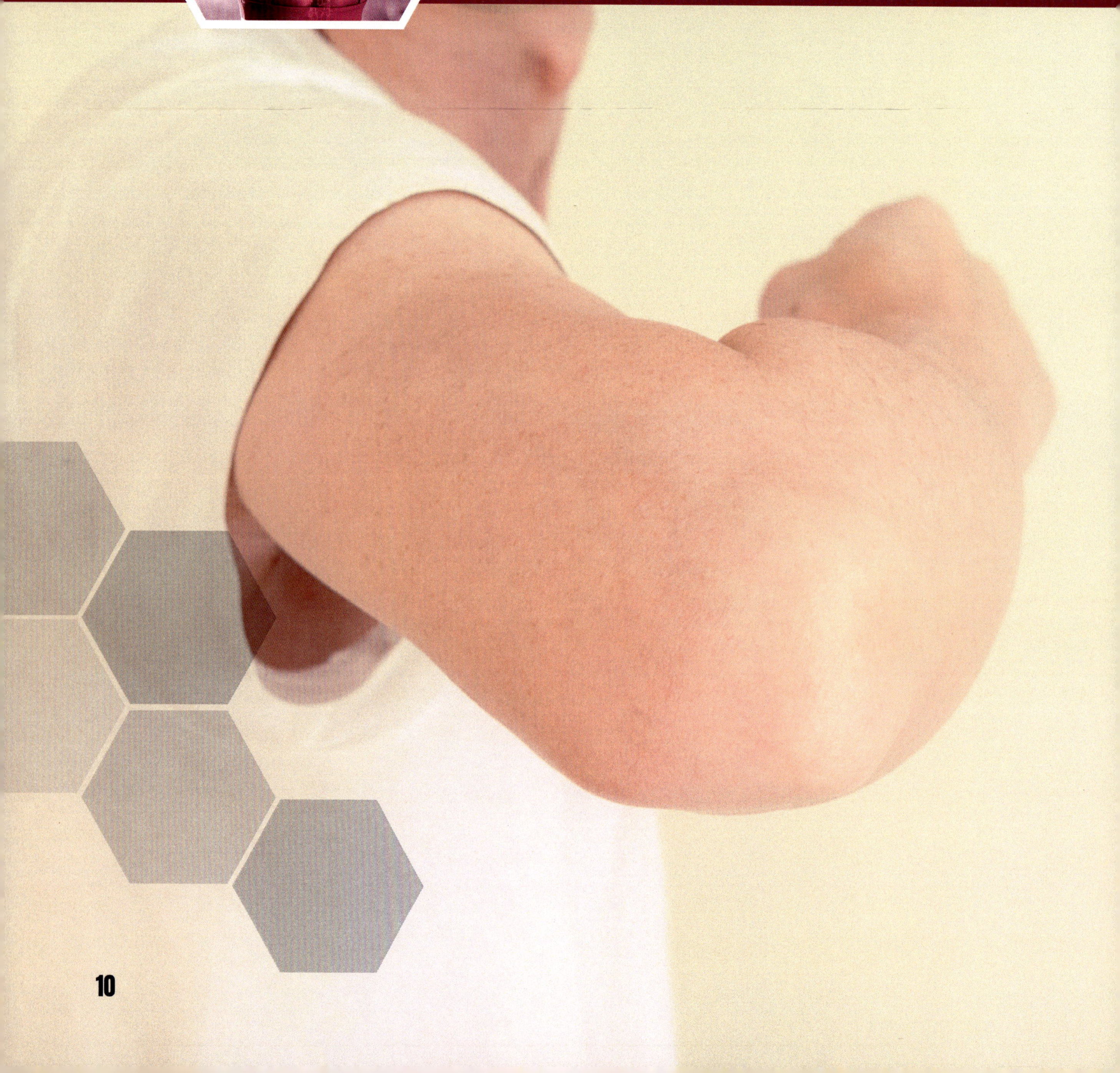

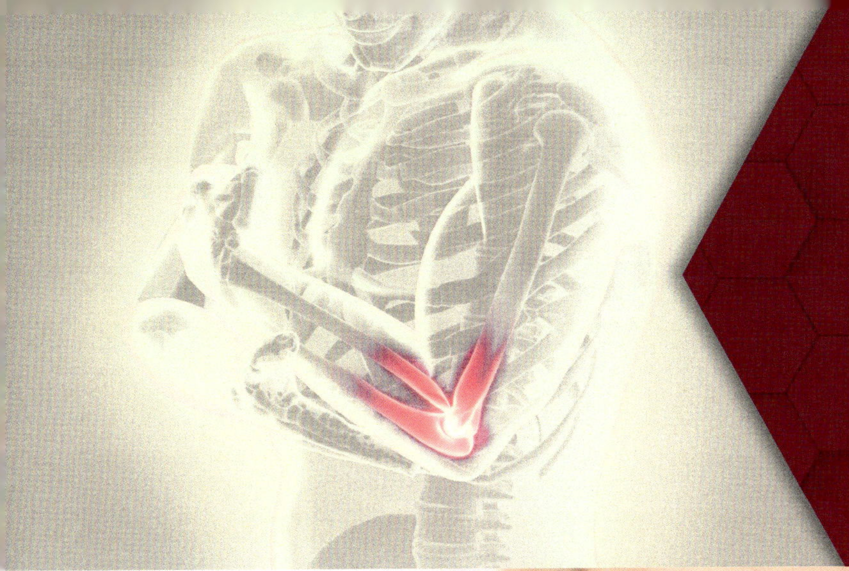

Your elbow is a mobile joint. It is where your humerus, radius, and ulna come together. Your elbow joint allows the lower arm to **extend** and **flex.** It also allows your lower arm to rotate clockwise and counterclockwise. Doctors and physical therapists call clockwise rotation **supination** and counterclockwise rotation **pronation.**

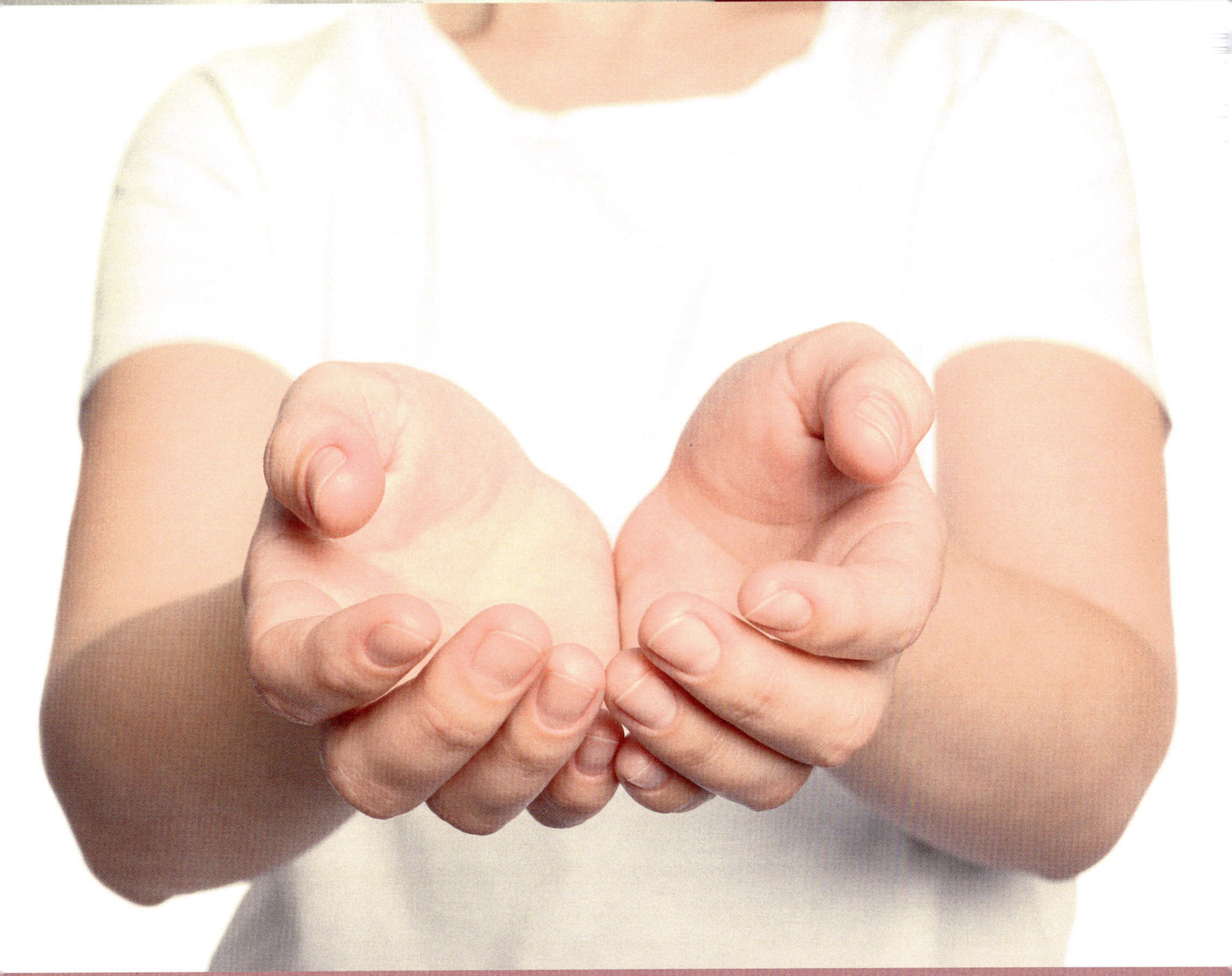

Pronation and supination are terms that refer to what direction a part of your body is turning. There's an easy way to remember which direction is supination for your arm. Hold your arm in front of you and then turn your arm so that your palm is facing upwards, like you could hold some soup in it. You've rotated using supination!

Ligaments

Ligaments are bands of tough, dense soft tissue that connect bones and organs to help hold them in place. Think of them like strong ropes. You have over 900 ligaments in your body! There are many ligaments in your elbow that connect your humerus to your radius and ulna and work to keep your upper and lower arms in place.

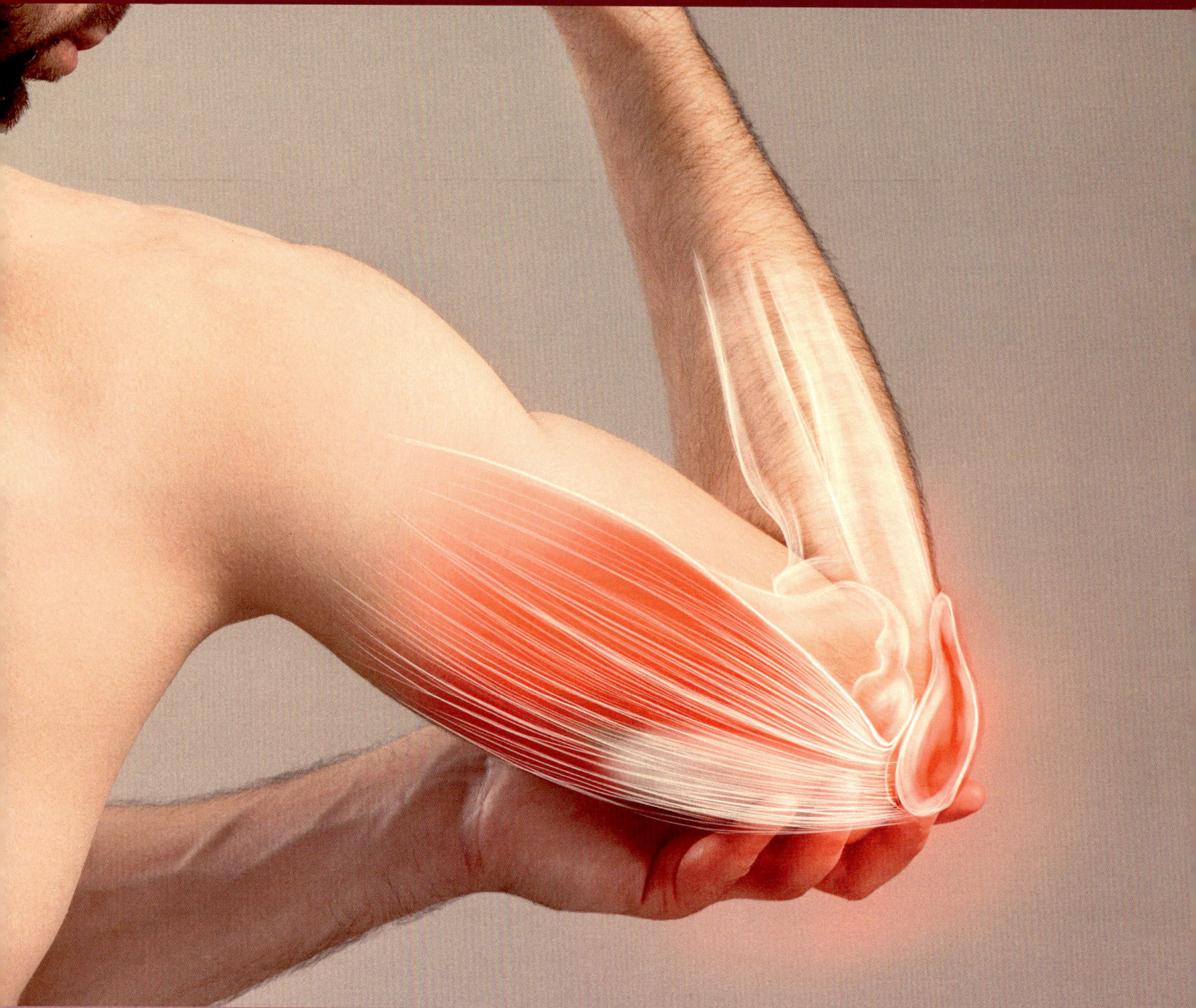

Sometimes people use the words "tendon" and "ligament" to mean the same thing, but they're actually different. Tendons connect muscle to bone. Ligaments connect bones to other bones.

Ulnar Collateral Ligament

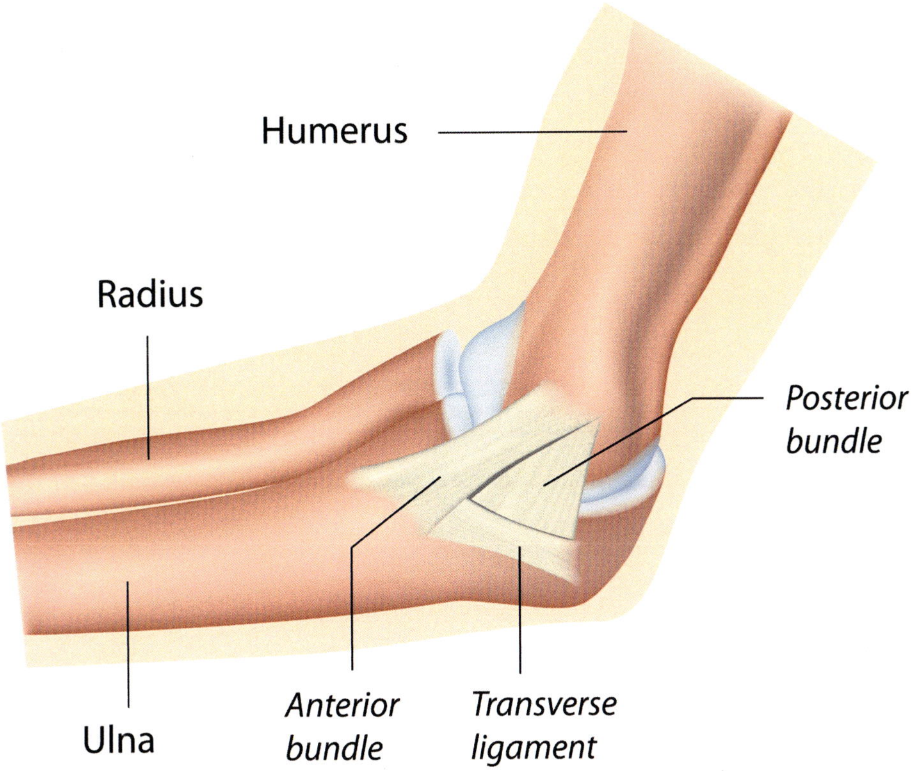

The ulnar collateral ligament (UCL) is an important ligament of your elbow. It runs from your humerus to the ulna. This ligament is on the inside, or pinky side, of your elbow. There are three bands of fibers that make up this ligament. The anterior band is in the front. This band is the most important for keeping your elbow stable.

Pitcher's elbow is a common name for a condition caused by a number of possible injuries. The most common is an injury to the UCL. This is the ligament that is strained or torn because of repetitive use.

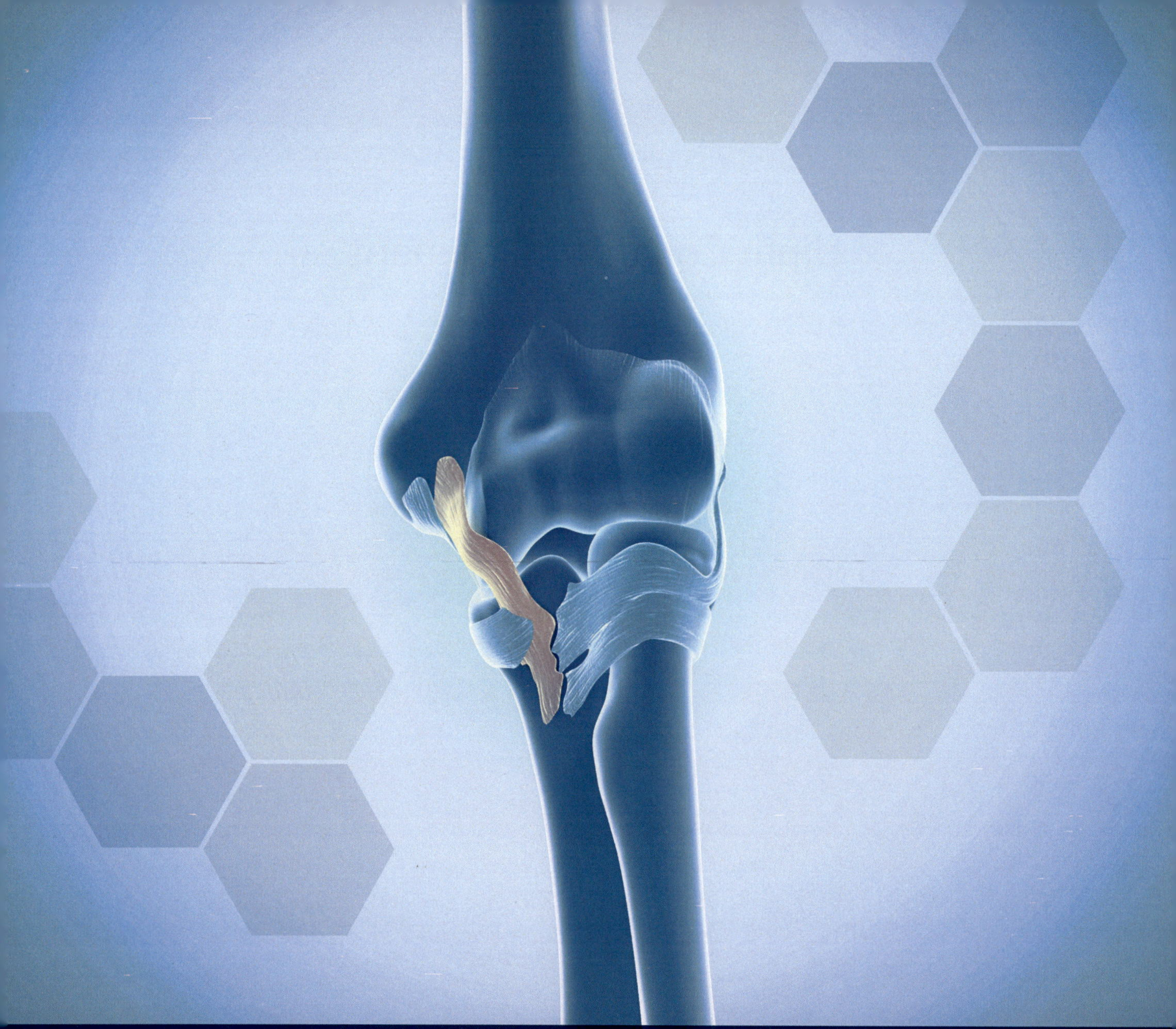

Chapter 3: Causes of Pitcher's Elbow

You get a pitcher's elbow injury when your ulnar collateral ligament (UCL) is stretched too far. UCL injuries are usually over-use injuries. This means that there isn't one specific moment when you're injured.

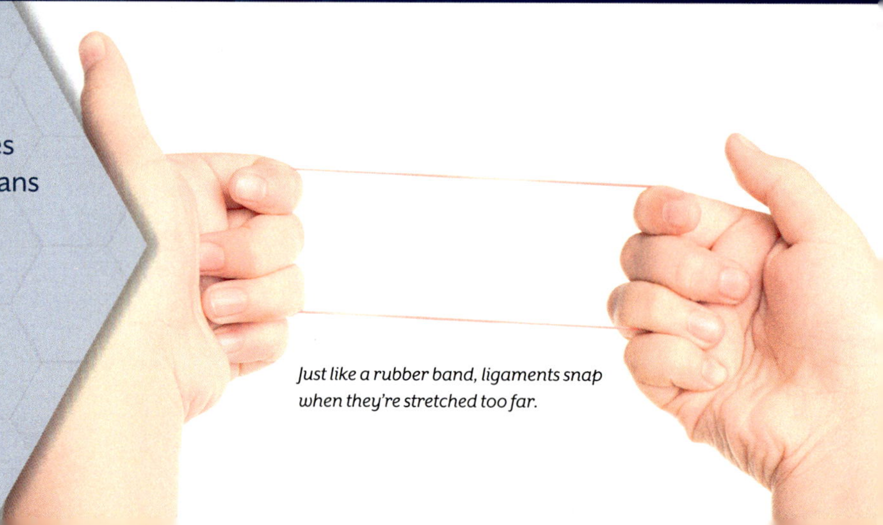

Just like a rubber band, ligaments snap when they're stretched too far.

Throwing is a complex motion. A pitcher's arm moves fast as it whips through the air. When scientists studied pitches, they found that a pitcher's arm can move 7,000 degrees per second. That's as fast as a tire rotates on a car going 93 miles per hour (153 kph)!

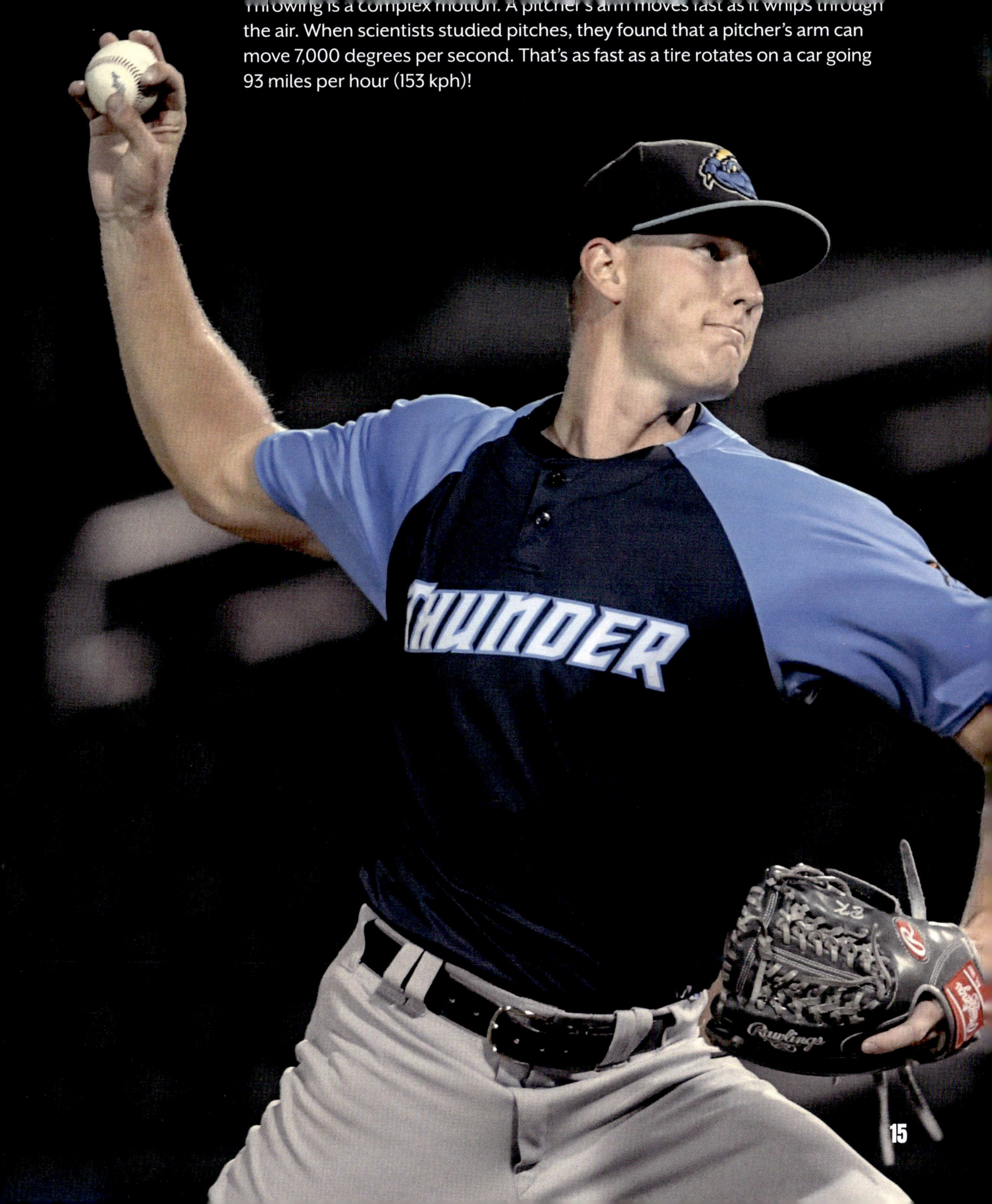

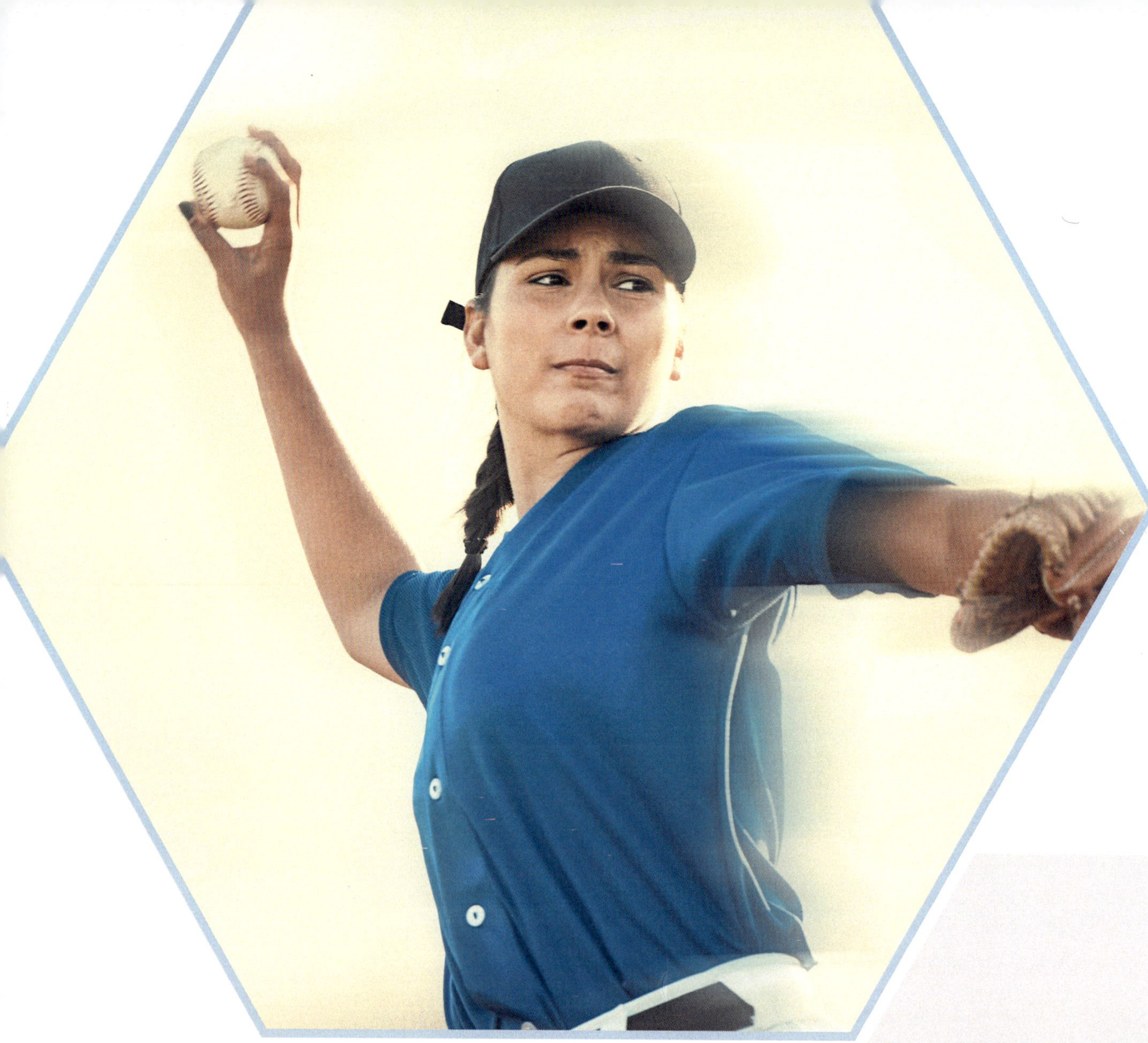

Throwing happens fast, but there are some parts of the motion that are more dangerous than others. The biggest chance for injury is when your arm is pulled backward all the way. As you bring your arm forward to throw a ball, the inside of your elbow experiences a high force. The UCL has to resist this force to keep the elbow stable.

During pitches, your UCL may experience a force of 60 pounds. That's like hanging 5 bowling balls off of your wrist. The muscles surrounding your elbow help protect it during throwing. Unfortunately, even with your muscles helping to protect your elbow, most of the load lands on your UCL.

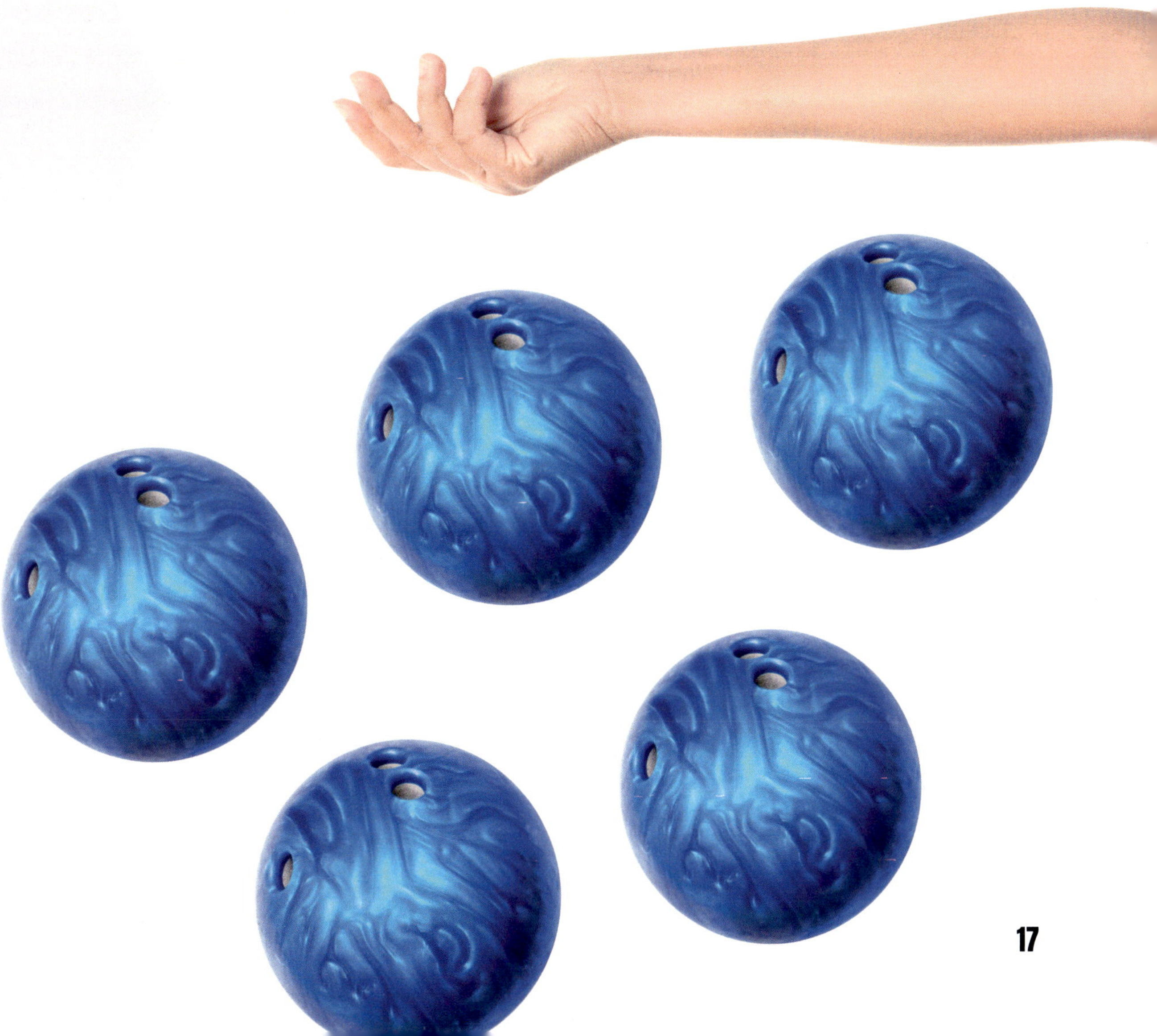

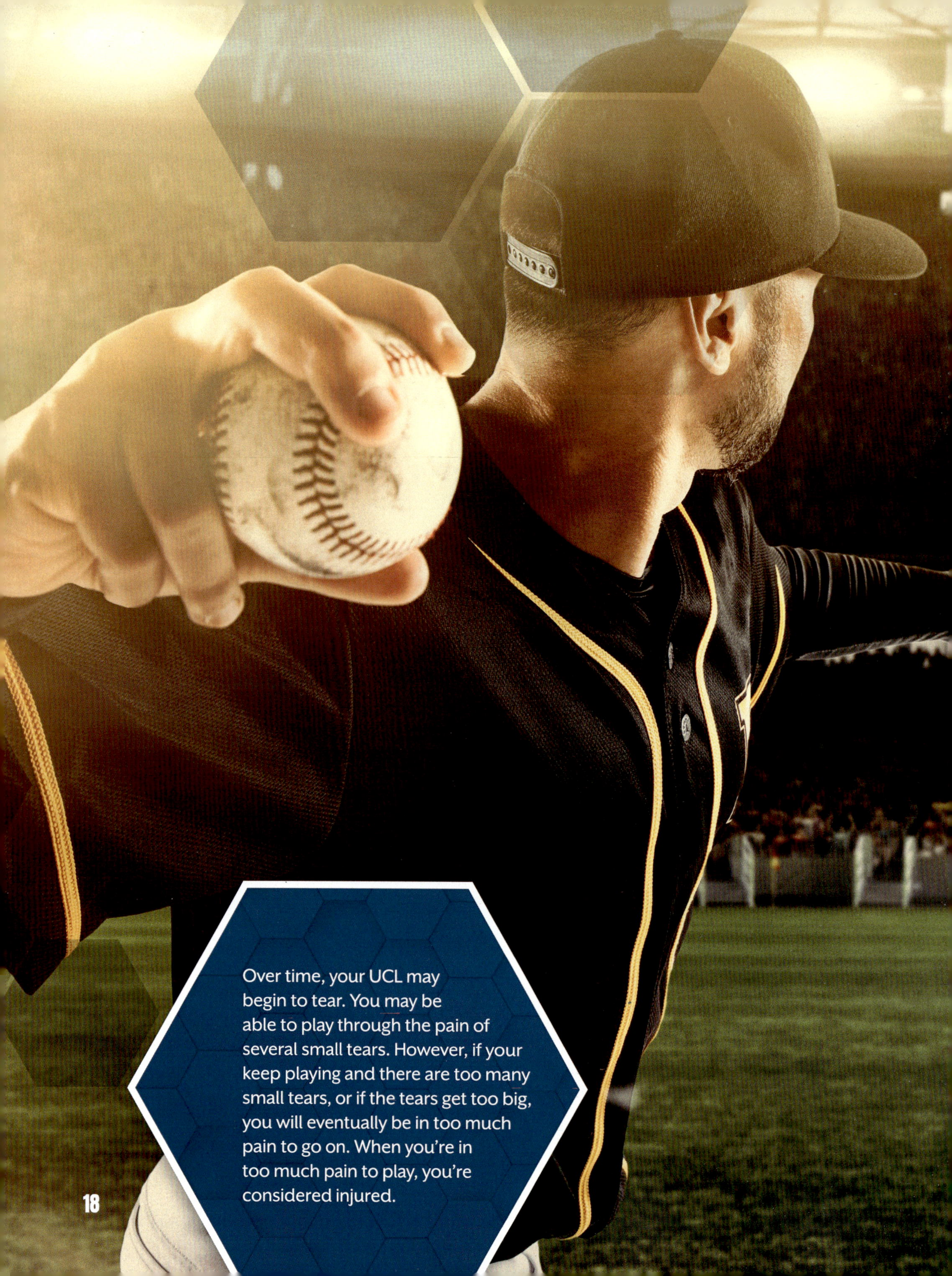

Over time, your UCL may begin to tear. You may be able to play through the pain of several small tears. However, if your keep playing and there are too many small tears, or if the tears get too big, you will eventually be in too much pain to go on. When you're in too much pain to play, you're considered injured.

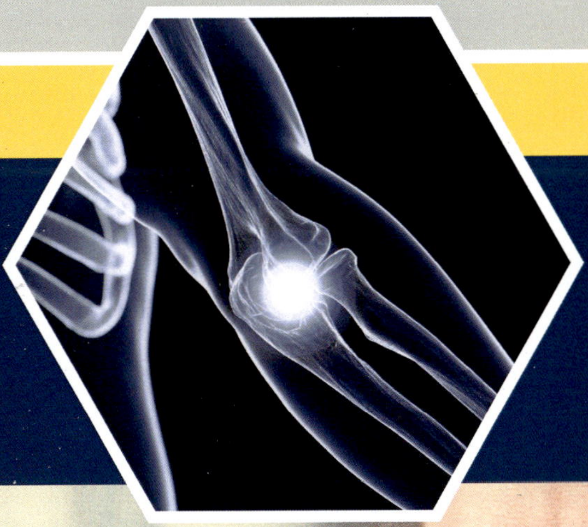

Sudden injury

Most UCL injuries happen slowly over time. Rarely, though, a UCL injury can happen all of a sudden. This is called an acute injury instead of an overuse injury. If this happens, you might feel a "pop" at your elbow followed by pain.

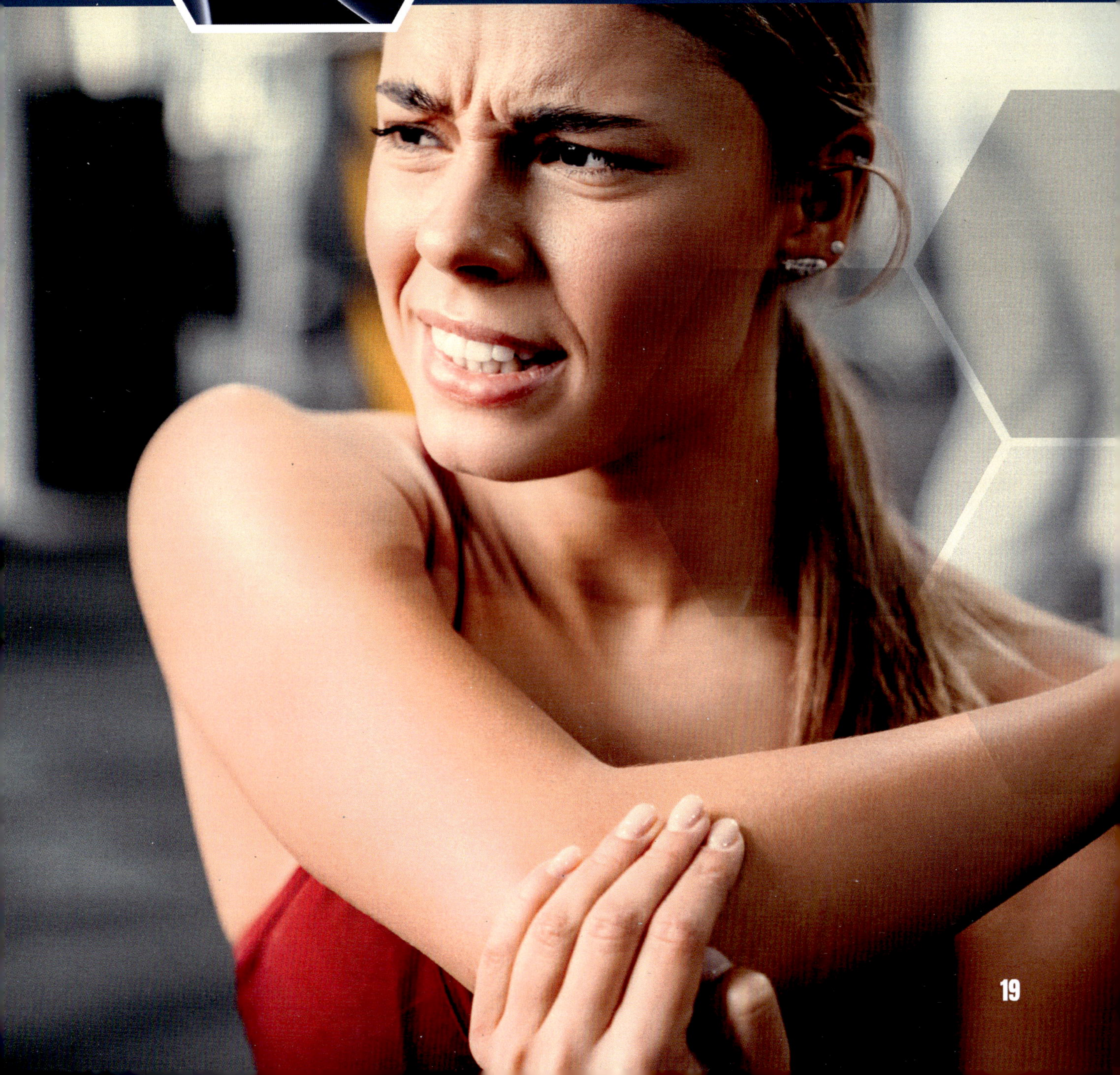

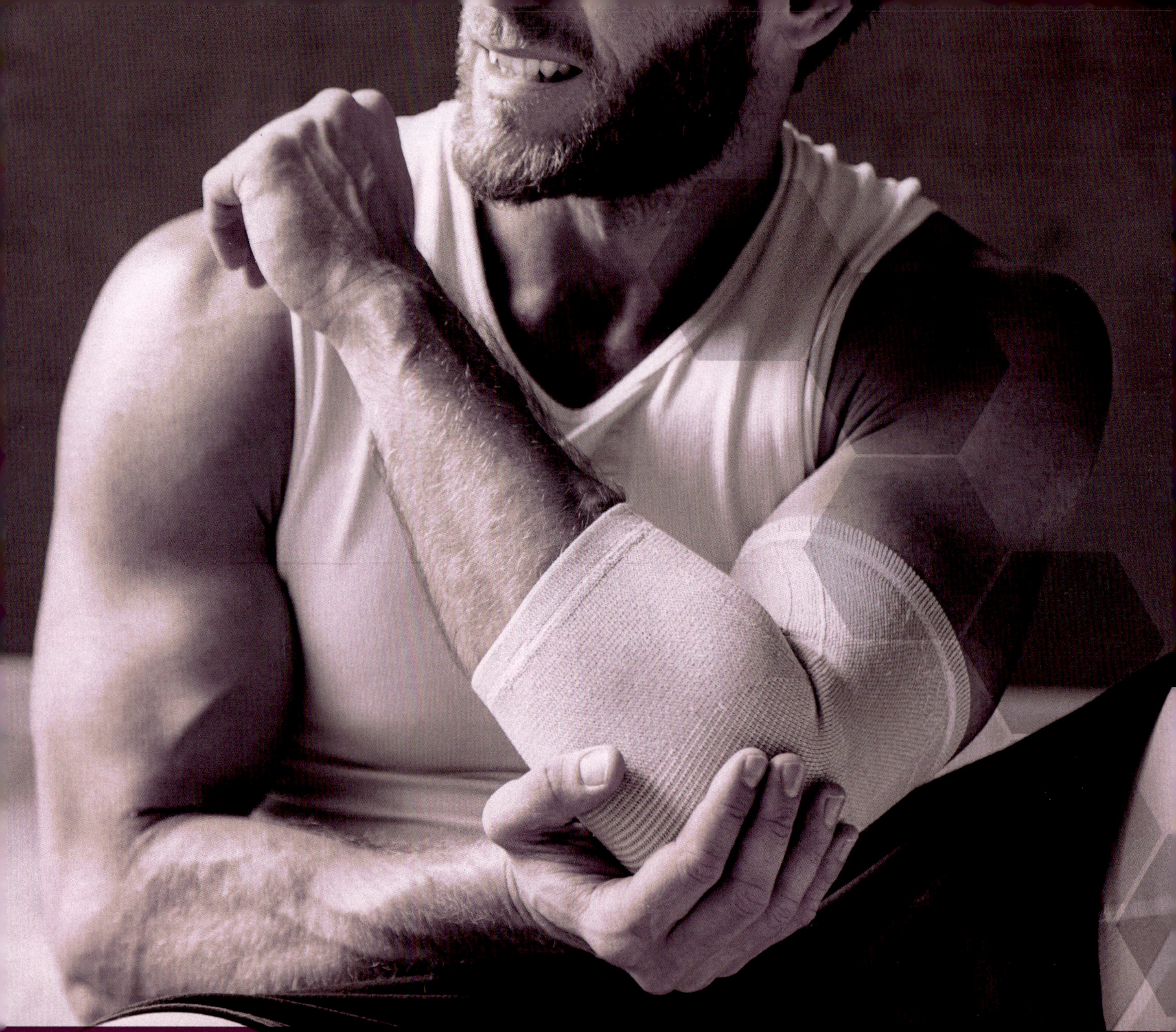

Chapter 4: Types of pitcher's elbow injuries

Pitcher's elbow injuries can range from just a small UCL strain to a complete tear. Doctors and medical professionals have developed a grading system to help identify how badly you're hurt. They use this grading system to recommend treatment.

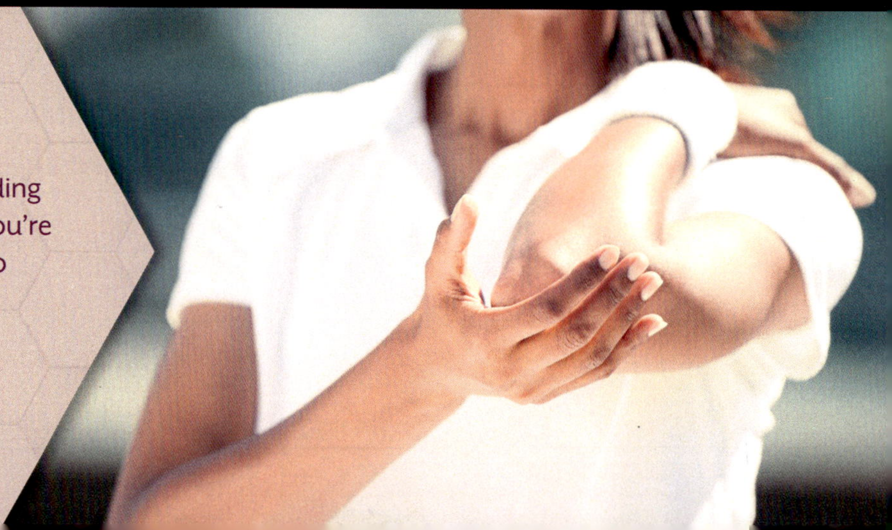

Grade 1

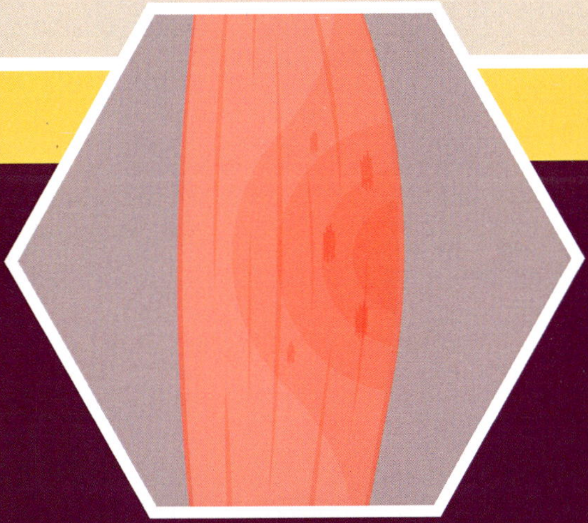

With a Grade 1 injury, your UCL is stretched but not torn.

Grade 2

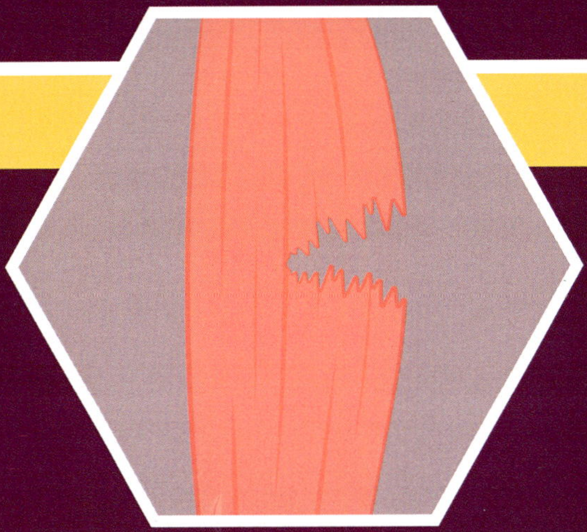

When you have a Grade 2 injury, your UCL will be stretched so that it is loose and partially torn.

Grade 3

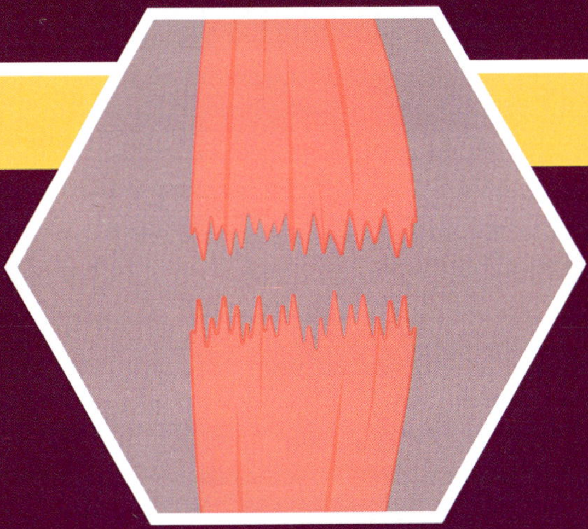

Grade 3 UCL injuries are the most severe. If your UCL is completely torn, then you have a Grade 3 injury.

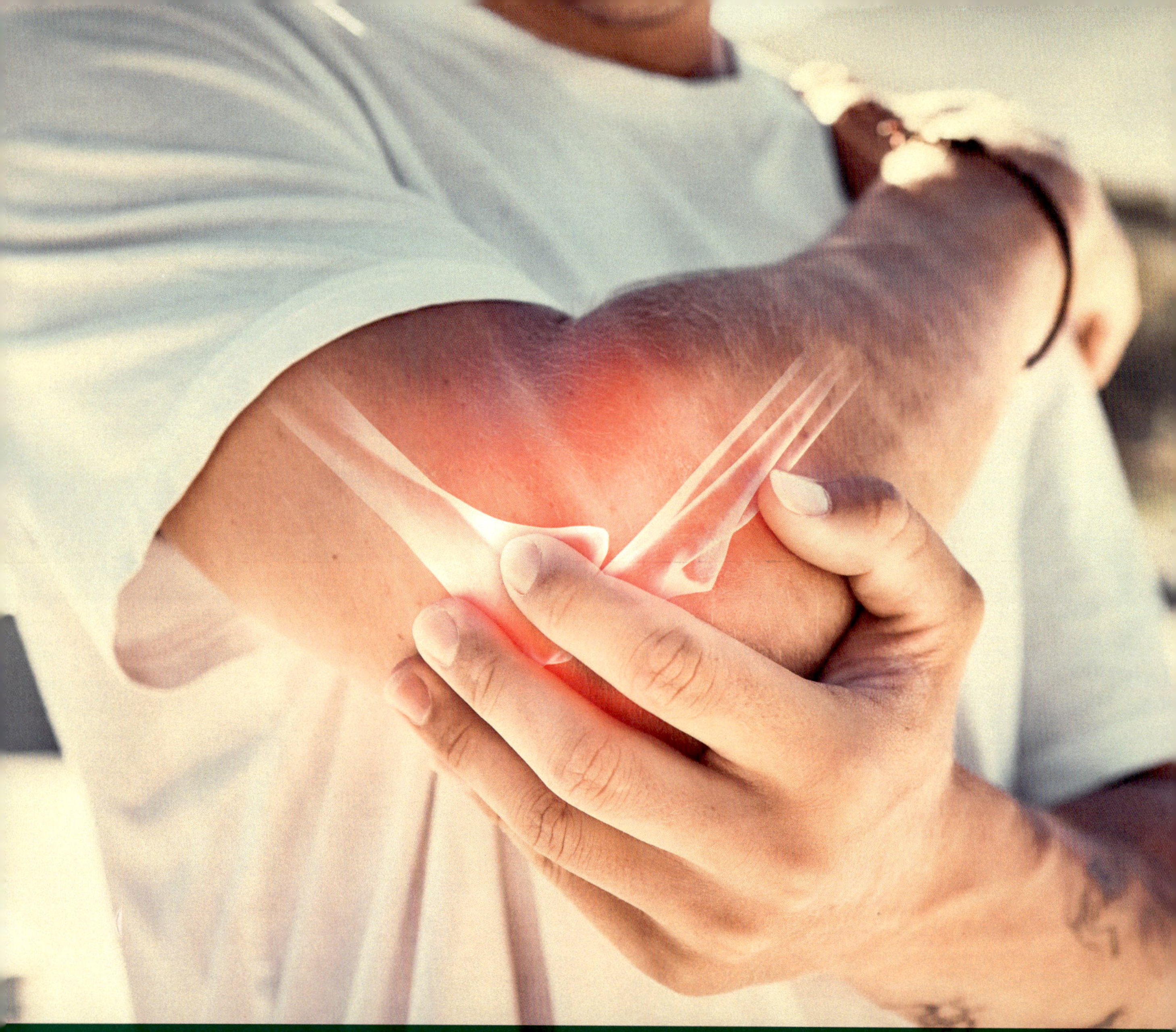

Chapter 5: Diagnosis

If you think you have any injury to your elbow, you should see a doctor, athletic trainer, or other medical professional. Pain in your elbow is one of the first signs you might have a UCL injury. Other signs include numbness at your fingertips and a loose feeling in your elbow. If you feel any of these signs, you should tell a coach, trainer, or doctor.

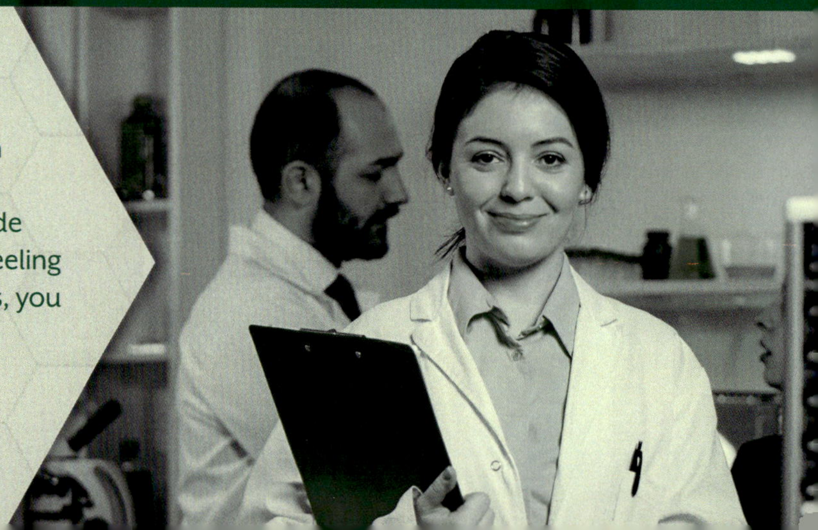

Doctors and trainers will ask you about your elbow. They will want to know when your pain started and how long it has gone on. If you think you have an injury that happened suddenly, they will want to know what you were doing when you heard a "pop" or felt pain.

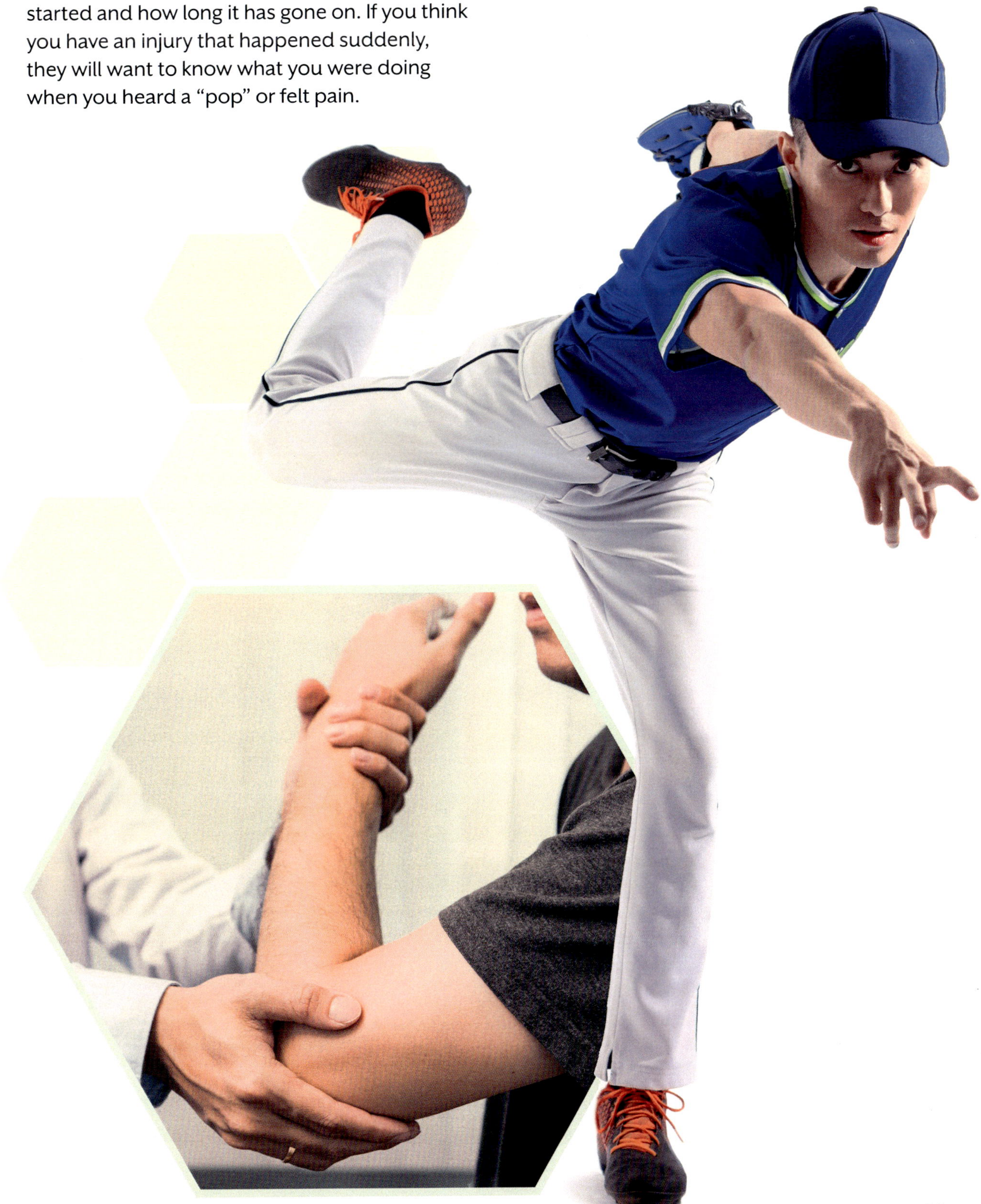

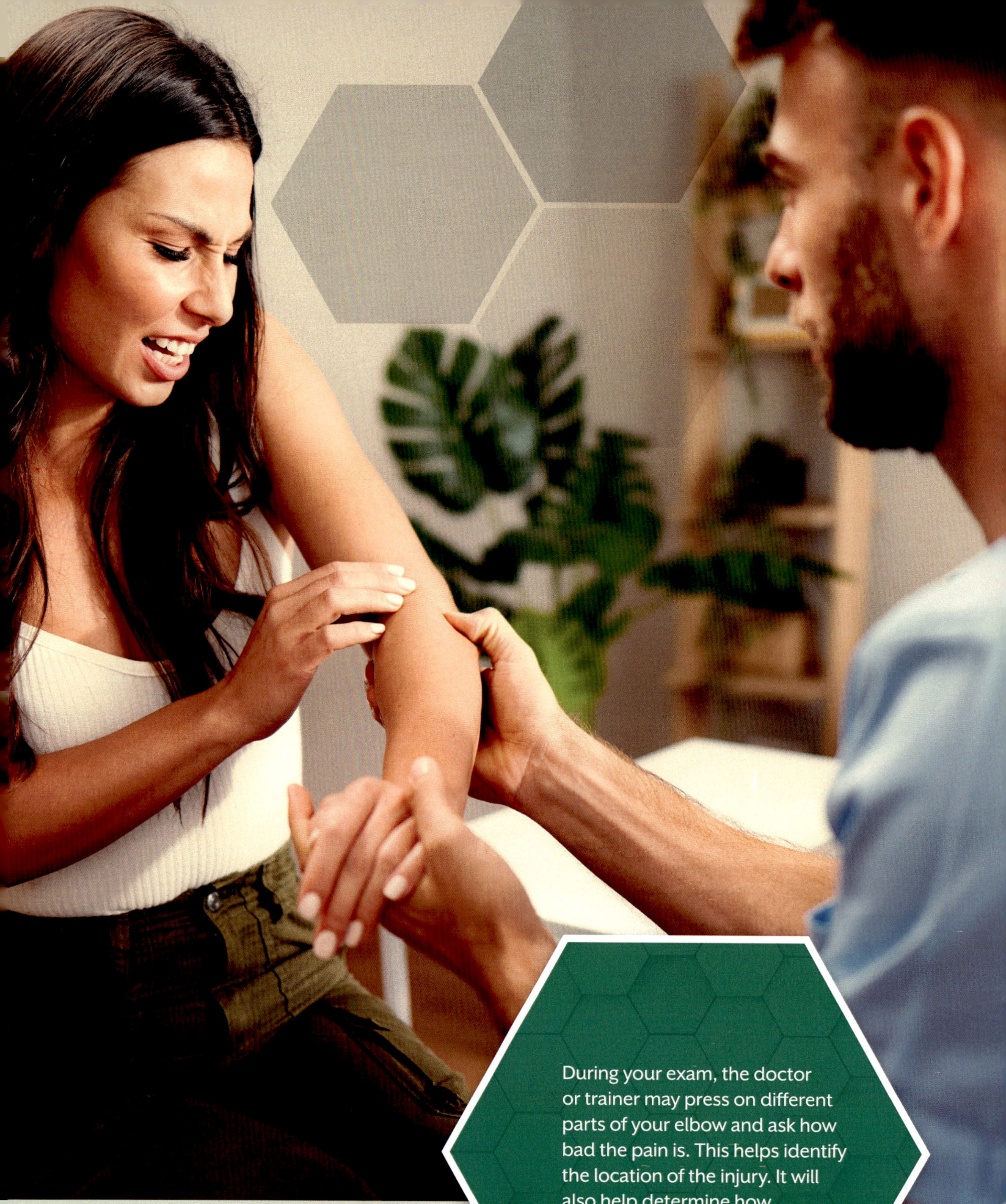

During your exam, the doctor or trainer may press on different parts of your elbow and ask how bad the pain is. This helps identify the location of the injury. It will also help determine how severely you're injured.

An important part of your exam will be comparing your injured arm to your uninjured arm. Range of motion is the name for how far your lower arm can move compared to your upper arm. If your injured arm has a different **range of motion** than your uninjured arm, that's a sign there is an injury. They will also compare the size and shape of your two elbow joints for muscle tone, bruising, and swelling.

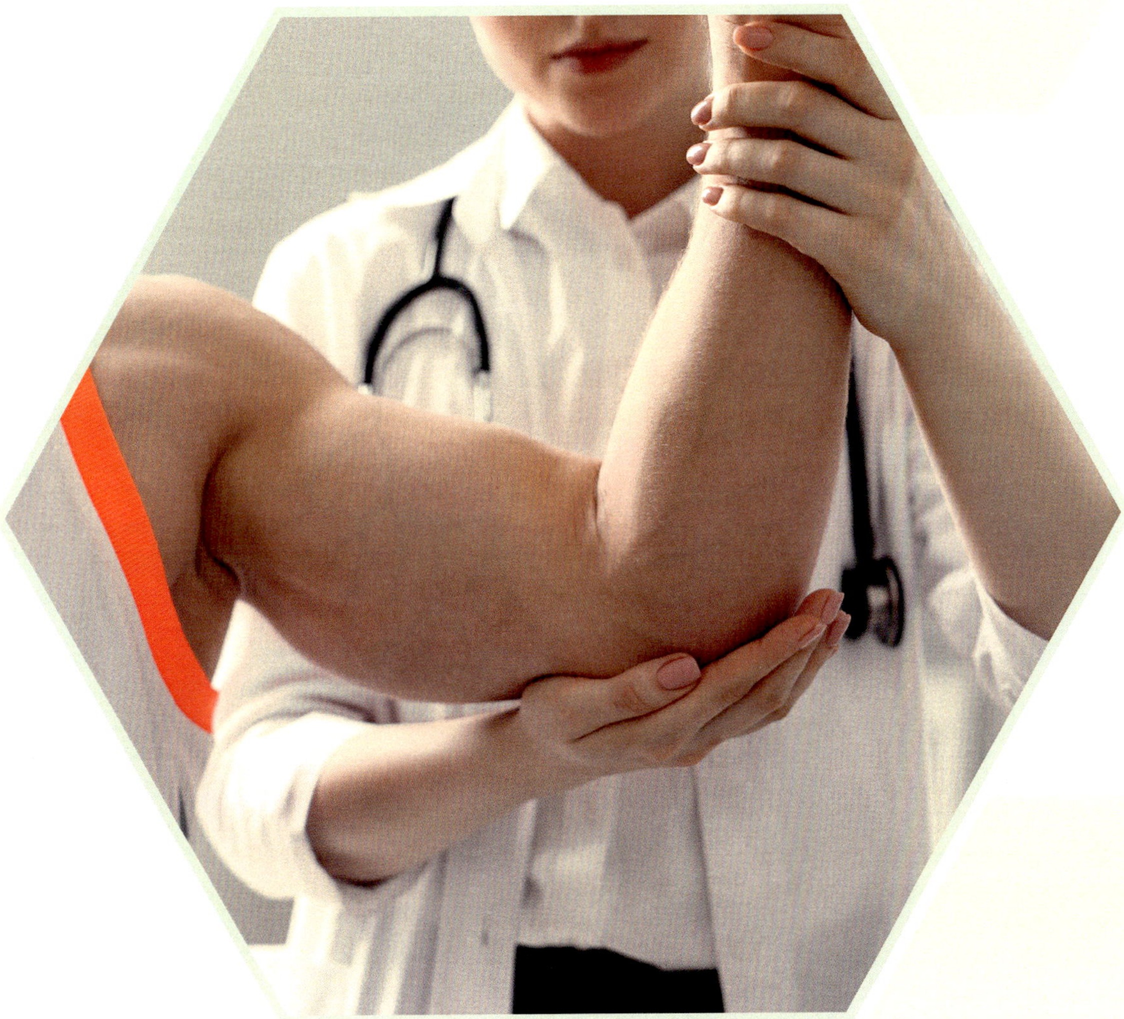

One test the doctor or trainer might perform is the **valgus stress test.** Valgus is a medical word that means away. In this test, a medical professional will move your lower arm away from your body while holding your upper arm in place.

If this motion causes pain, or if your arm moves more than it should, then you probably have a pitcher's elbow injury.

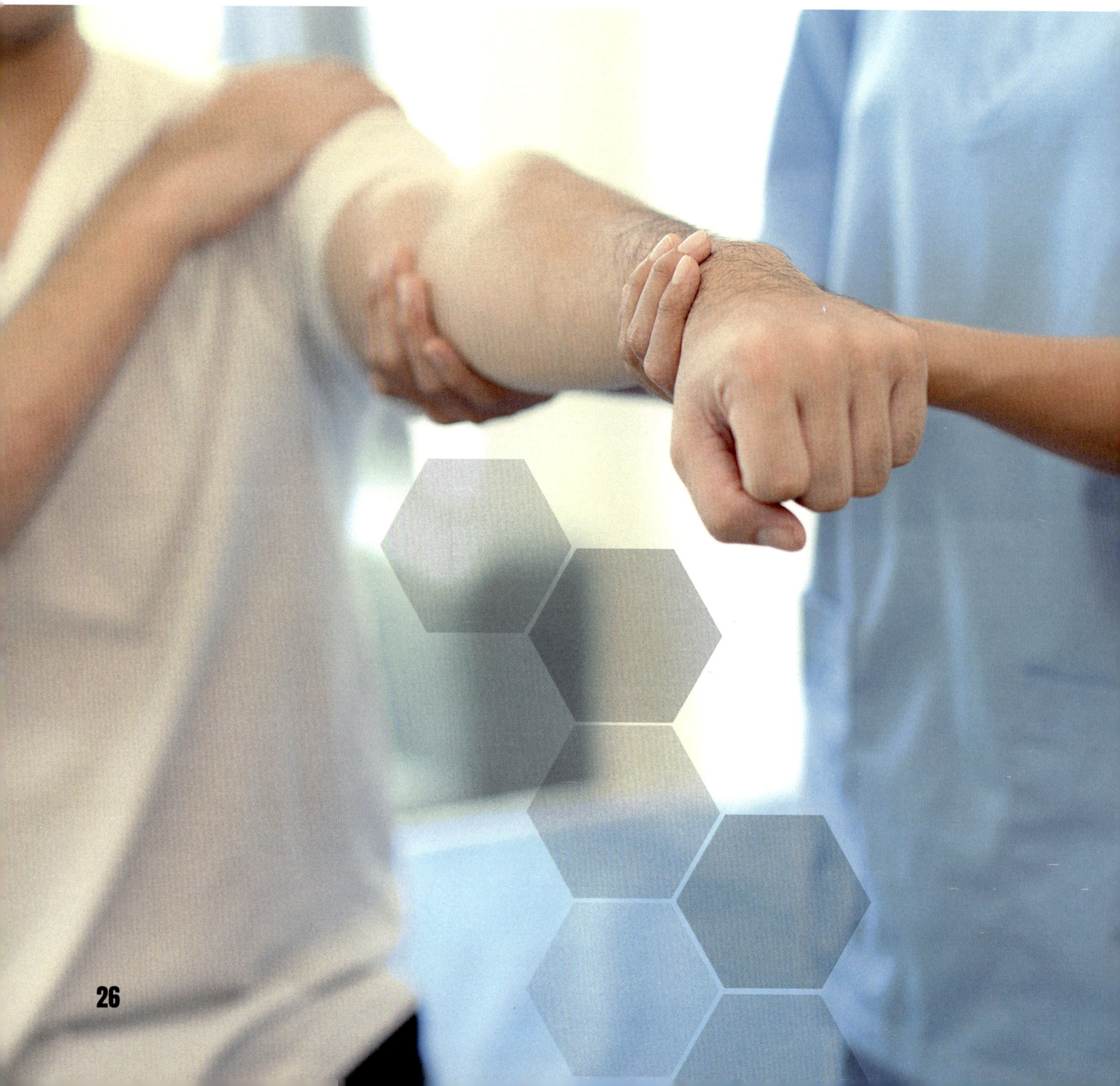

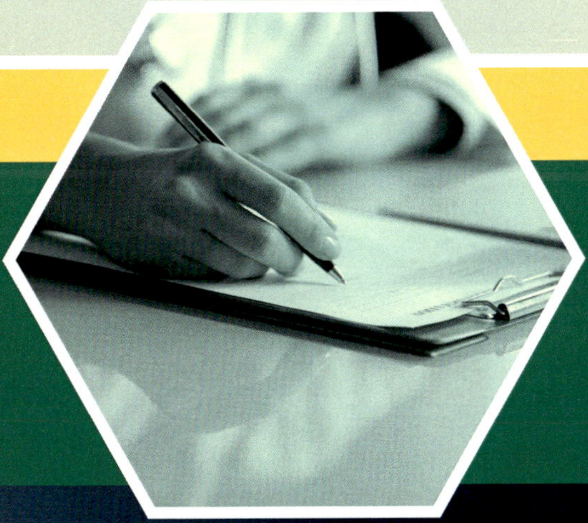

Imaging

There are many ways of seeing inside your body, and your doctor may order several tests to help determine how badly your UCL has been torn or stretched. This can help determine what type of treatment is best for your injury.

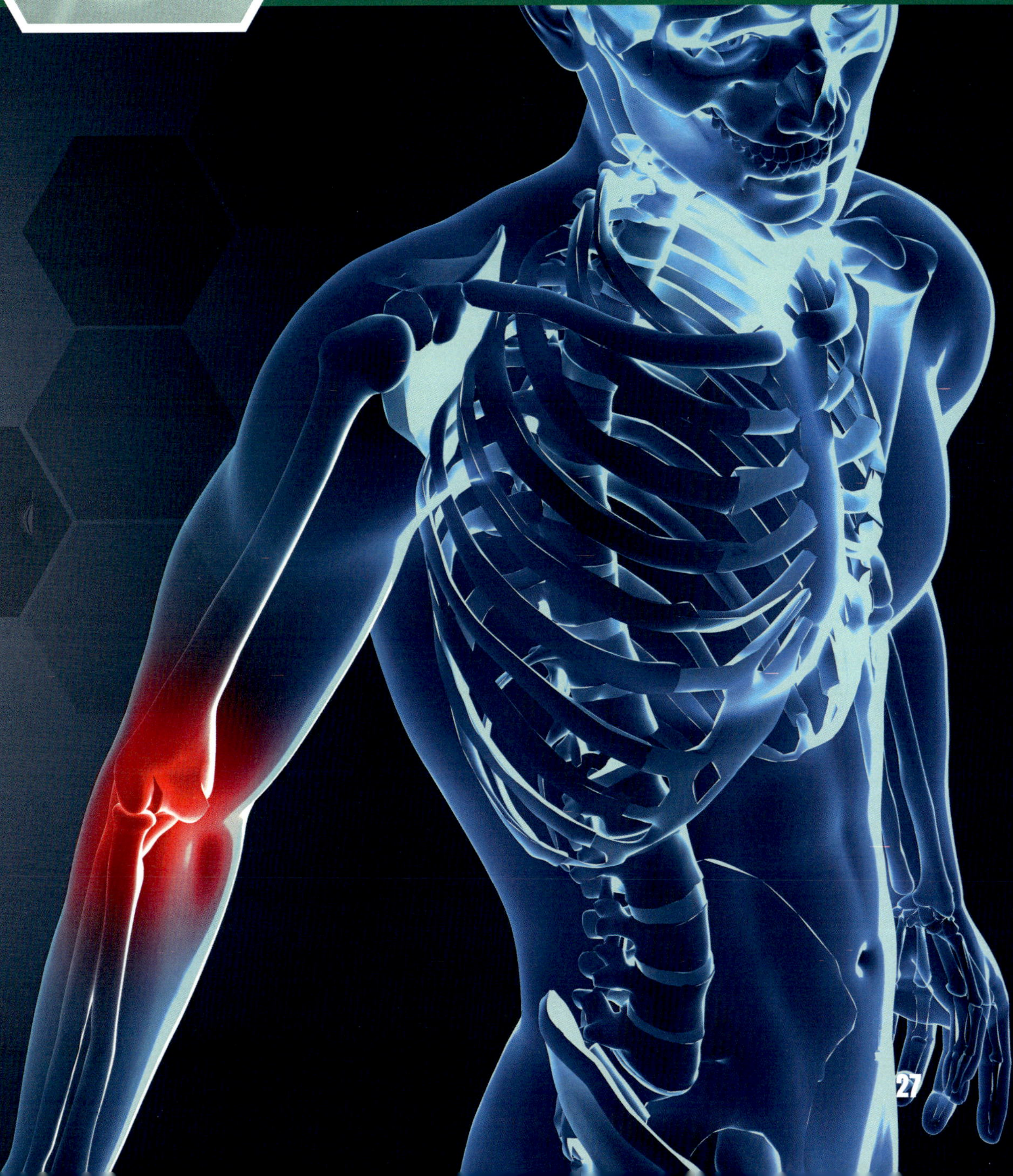

Magnetic Resonance Imaging, commonly called MRI, is used to look at your muscle and soft tissue. An MRI uses radio waves produced by a computer and a strong magnetic field to create imagines of the inside of your body. This can help doctors find out the amount of tear in your UCL.

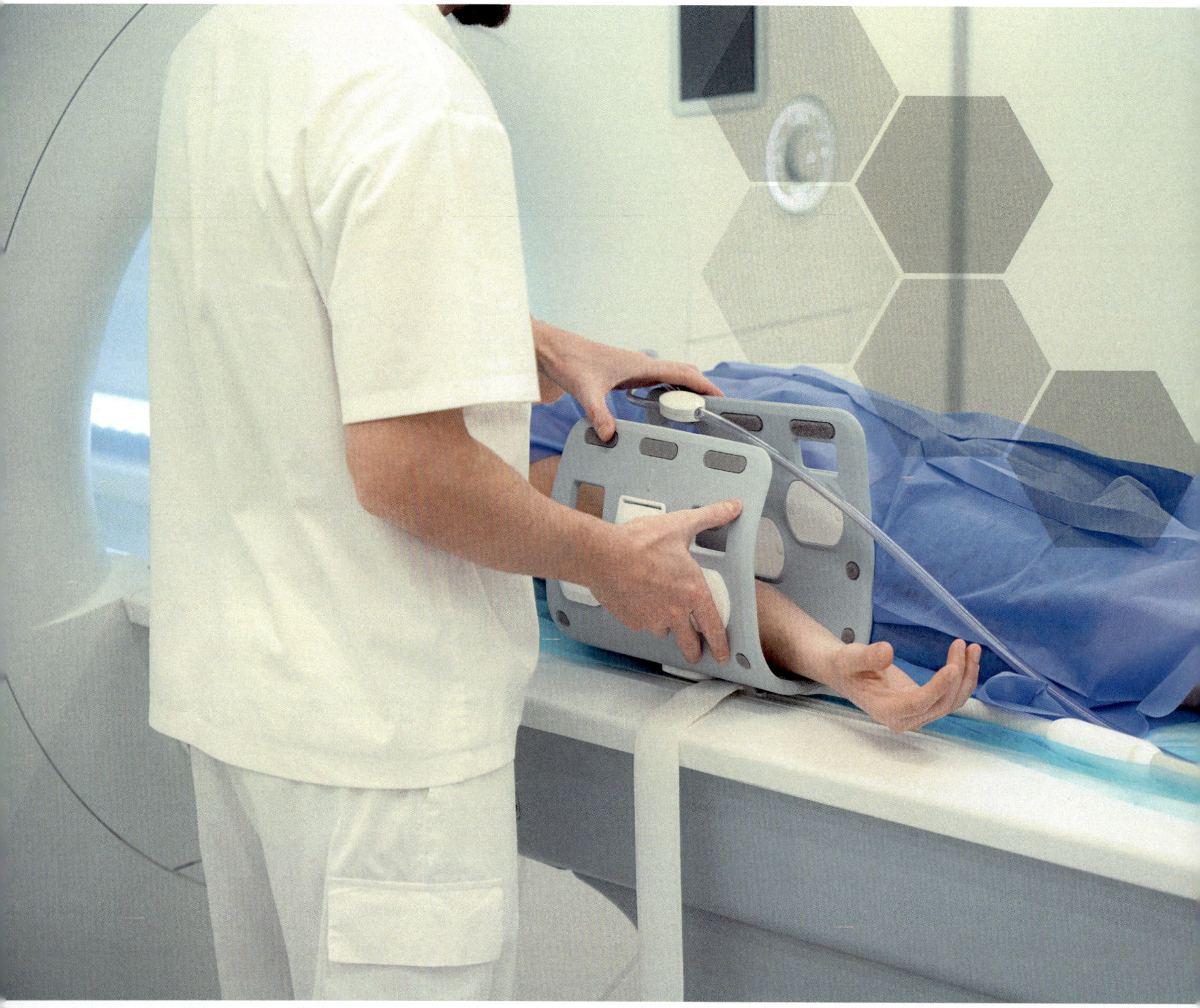

The idea for MRI machines has been around since the 1930s. However, it took about 40 years to make a working MRI machine. The first successful MRI scan of a human took place in 1977.

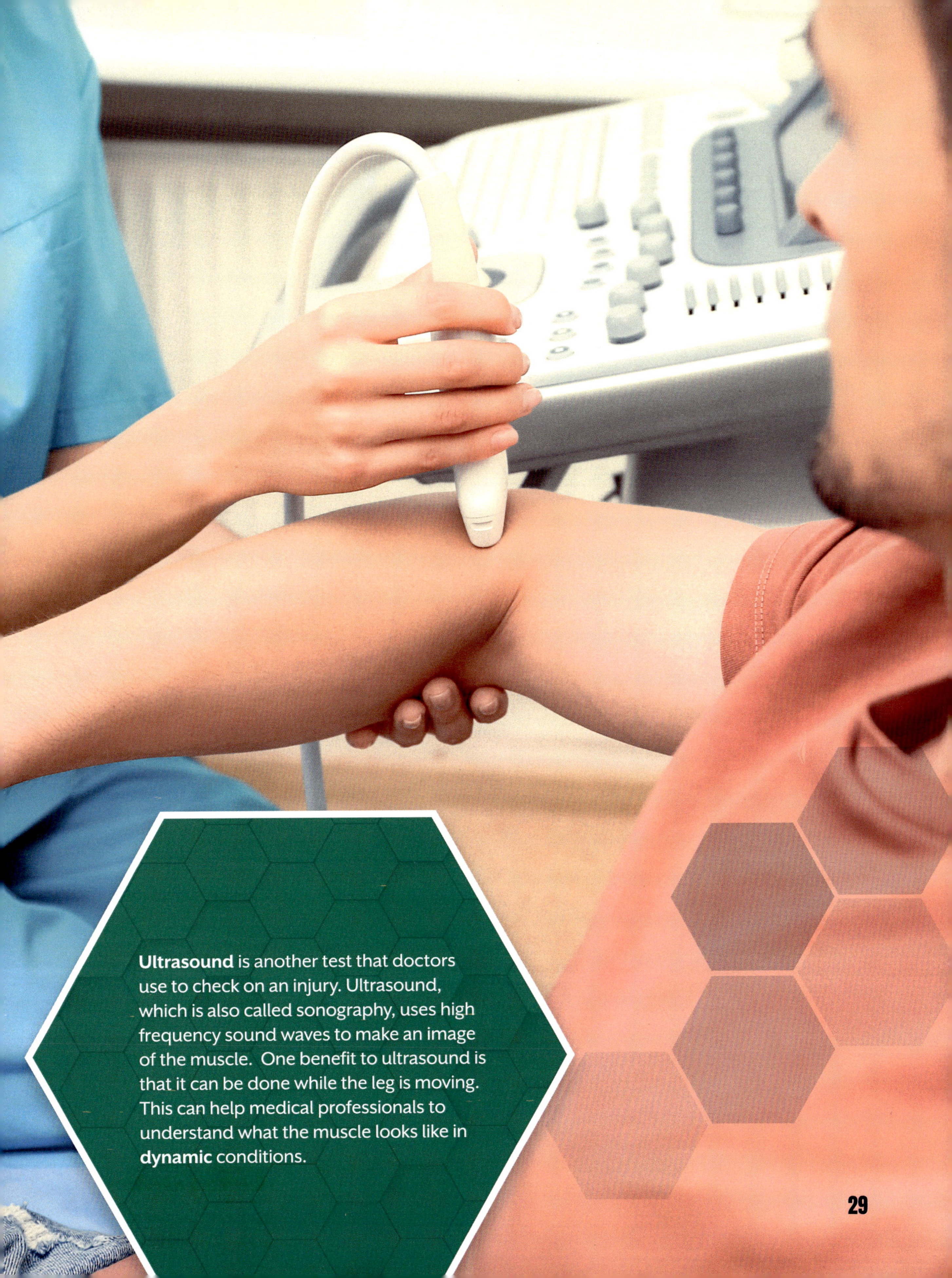

Ultrasound is another test that doctors use to check on an injury. Ultrasound, which is also called sonography, uses high frequency sound waves to make an image of the muscle. One benefit to ultrasound is that it can be done while the leg is moving. This can help medical professionals to understand what the muscle looks like in **dynamic** conditions.

In rare cases, a piece of bone may have torn away when your ligament was injured. When this happens, it's called an avulsion injury. This is more likely with UCL injuries that happened suddenly rather than with overuse injuries.

If doctors think an avulsion injury may have occurred, they can order an X-ray. X-rays take pictures of bone but don't show any muscle or other soft tissue like tendons. Doctors use these images to see if parts of your bone have been removed during an avulsion injury.

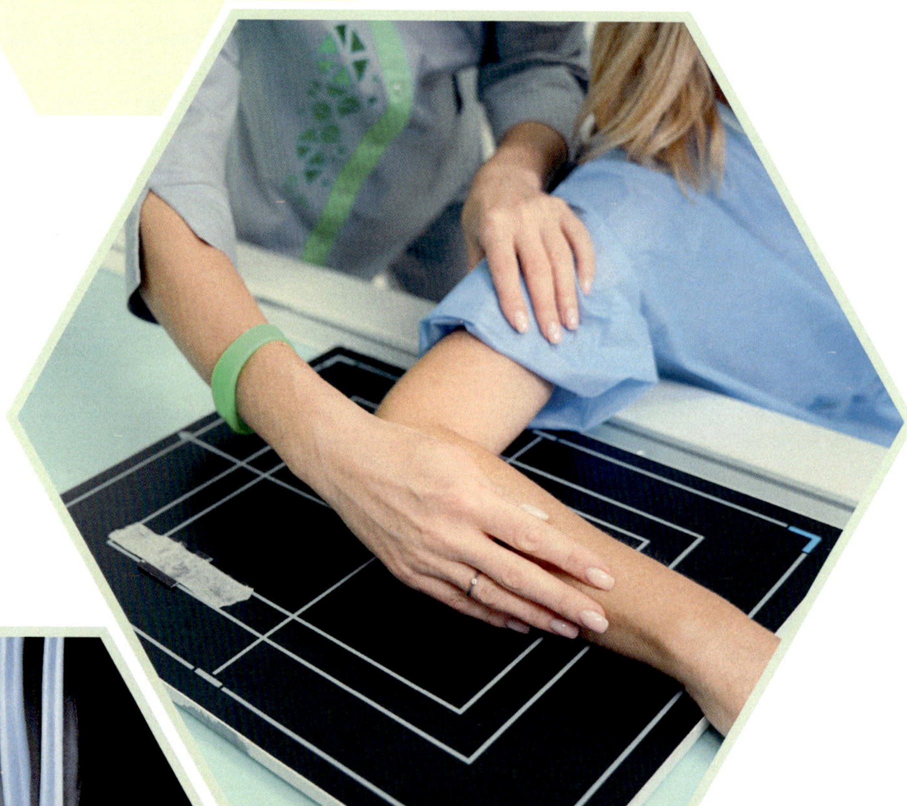

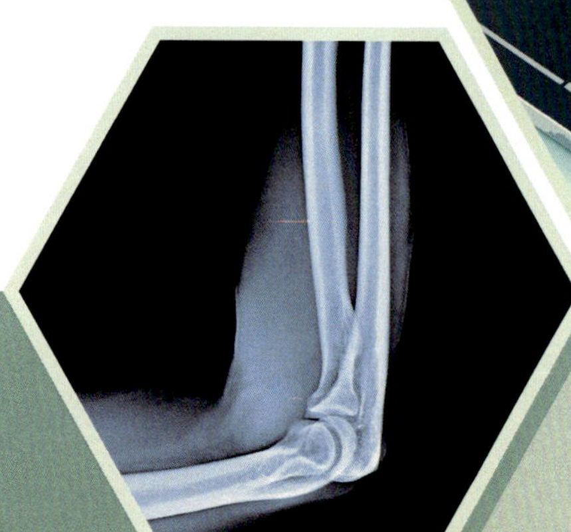

X-rays were discovered by accident in 1895, but they quickly were shown to be useful in a lot of places, including medicine. Wilhelm Roentgen was given the first Nobel Prize in physics in 1901 for his discovery of X-rays.

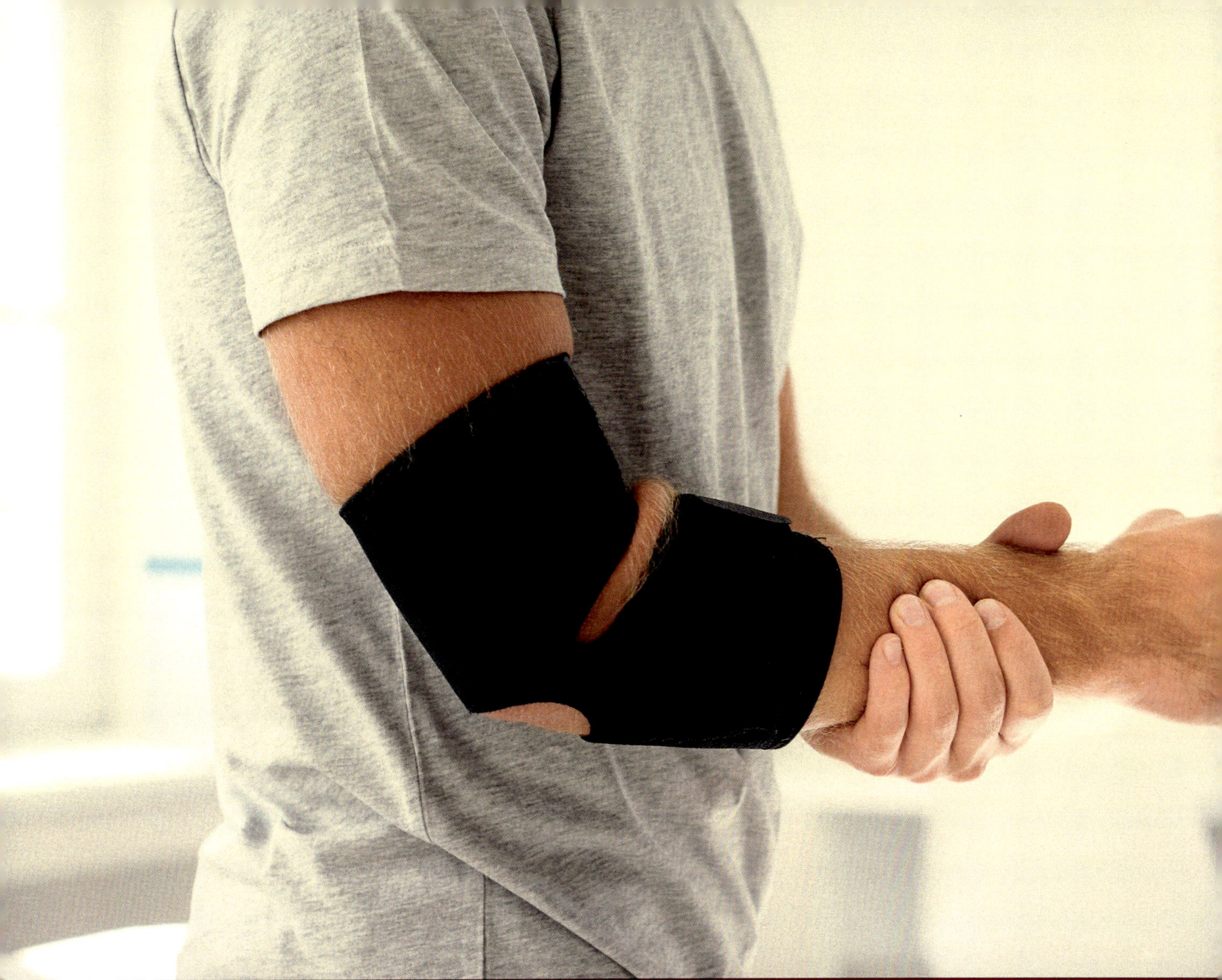

Chapter 6: Treatment

There are many ways to treat pitcher's elbow. Your doctor will recommend a treatment plan based on what grade of injury you have. No matter what the treatment is, it's important to follow all the directions and not return to play until the doctor say you're ready.

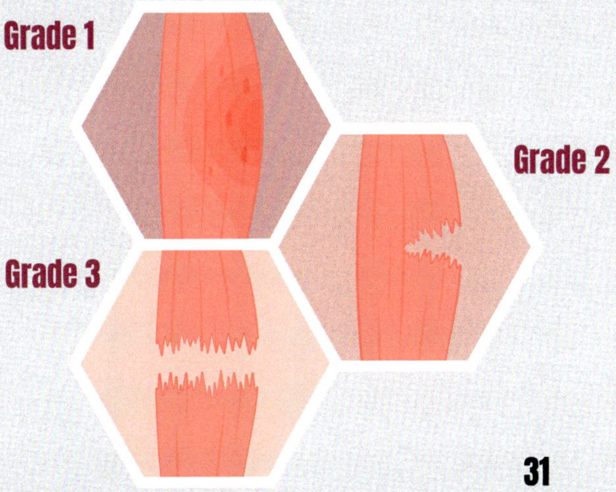

Non-surgical treatment

If you have a Grade 1 injury, you may recover without surgery. Your doctor or trainer may say that taking time away from playing sports and RICE will help you heal. RICE stands for

- Rest
- Ice
- Compression
- Elevation

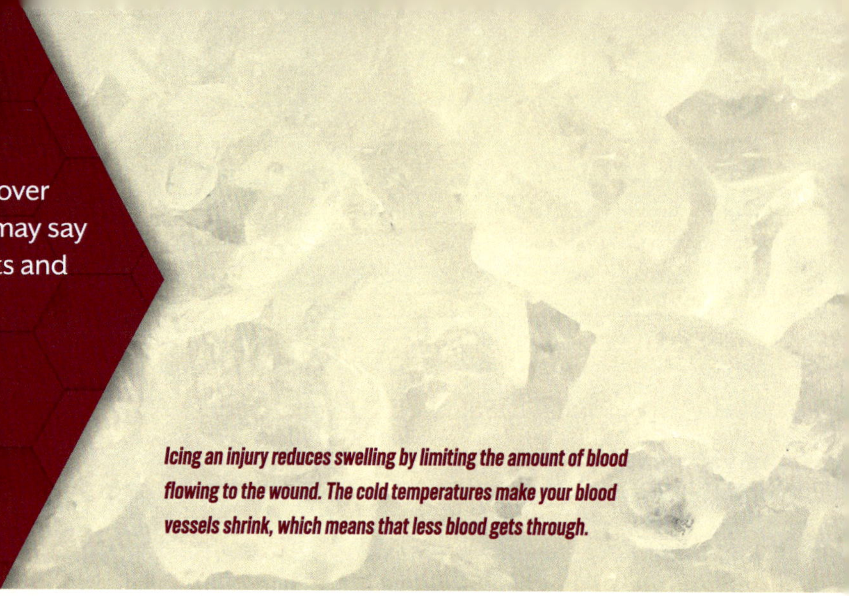

Icing an injury reduces swelling by limiting the amount of blood flowing to the wound. The cold temperatures make your blood vessels shrink, which means that less blood gets through.

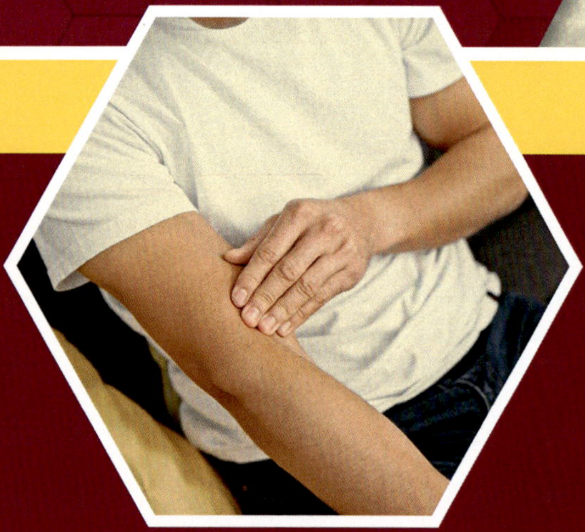

Rest

It is important to stop using your injured arm. You should not try to play sports while hurt.

Ice

Ice helps to keep swelling down and to decrease pain in the injured area. You should wrap ice packs in a cloth, rather than applying ice directly to your skin. After applying the ice for 20 minutes, wait at least 20 minutes before applying it again.

If your doctor tells you to ice an injury, they will also tell you how many times to apply the ice. Be sure to listen to your doctor's instructions so that you don't make the injury worse.

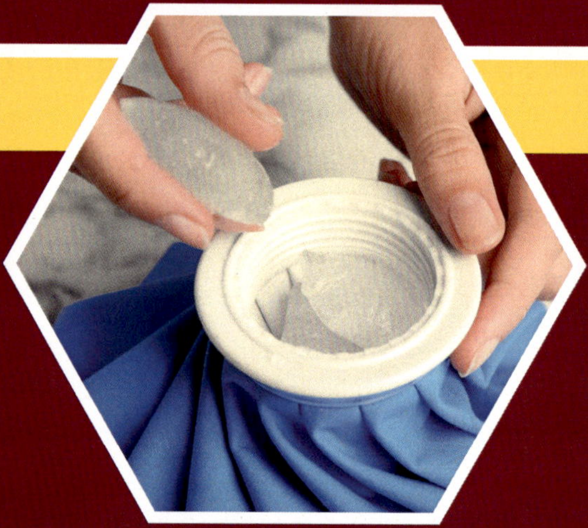

You can make an ice pack by combining 2 cups of water with 1 cup of rubbing alcohol or dish soap. Mix these together in a freezer bag, and place in the freezer for at least 1 hour.

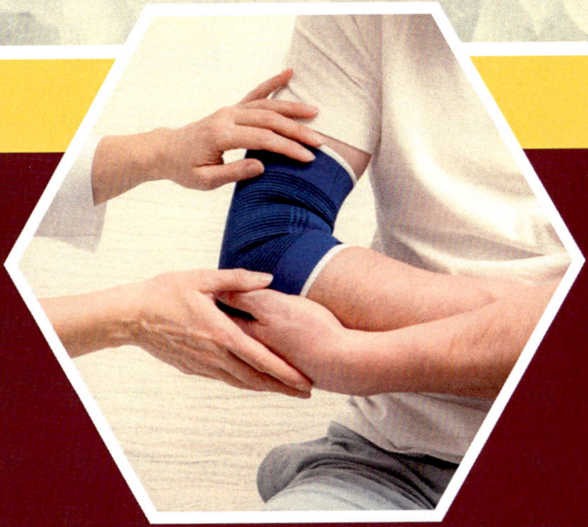

Compression

You may be given instructions to **compress** your injured elbow. Compression helps to decrease swelling. Your doctor or trainer may show you how to wrap your elbow with an elastic bandage.

Elevation

Elevating the injured limb means raising it higher than your heart. For a pitcher's elbow injury, this means that you should raise your elbow so that it's above your chest. Elevating the injury helps decrease swelling.

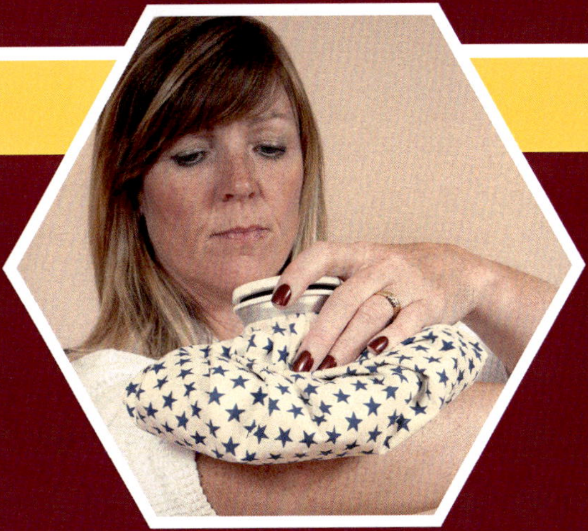

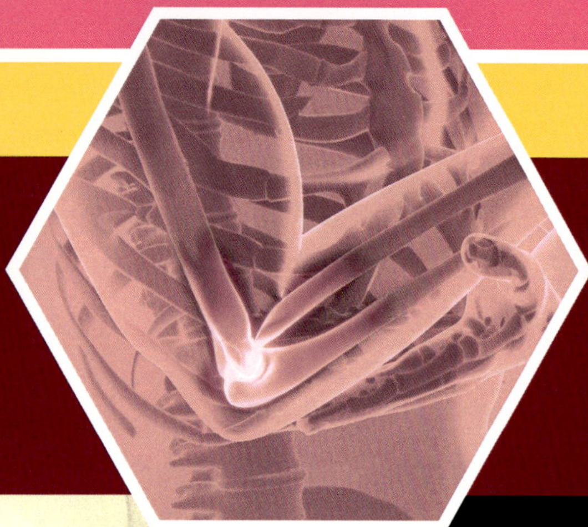

Tommy John Surgery

If your UCL is torn, then treating the injury with RICE won't be enough to heal it. Your doctor will likely recommend surgery. UCL replacement surgery is called a Tommy John surgery. MLB pitcher Tommy John's career was saved by the elbow surgery.

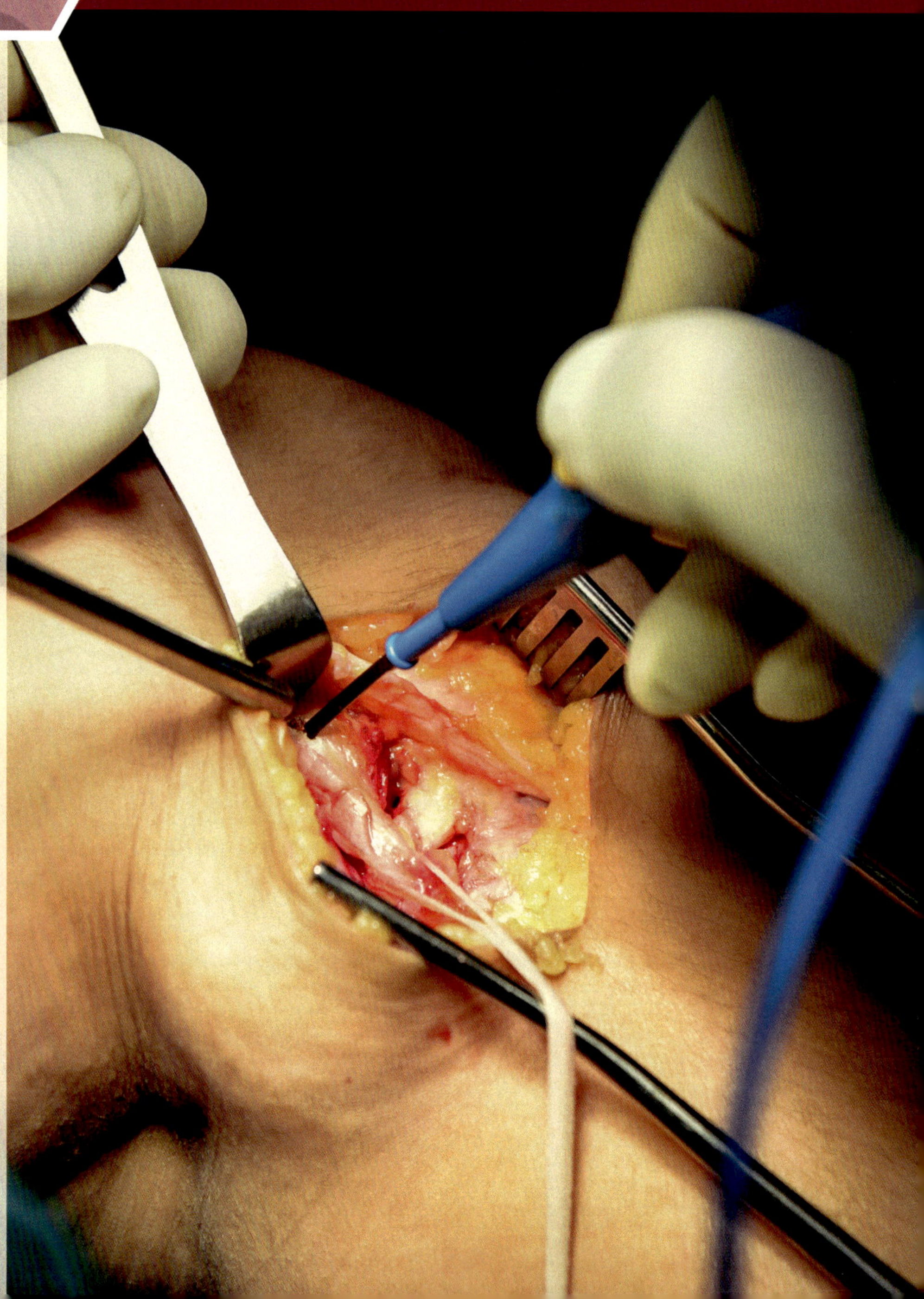

The first Tommy John surgery was performed in September, 1974. Tommy John recovered and went back to playing baseball in April, 1976.

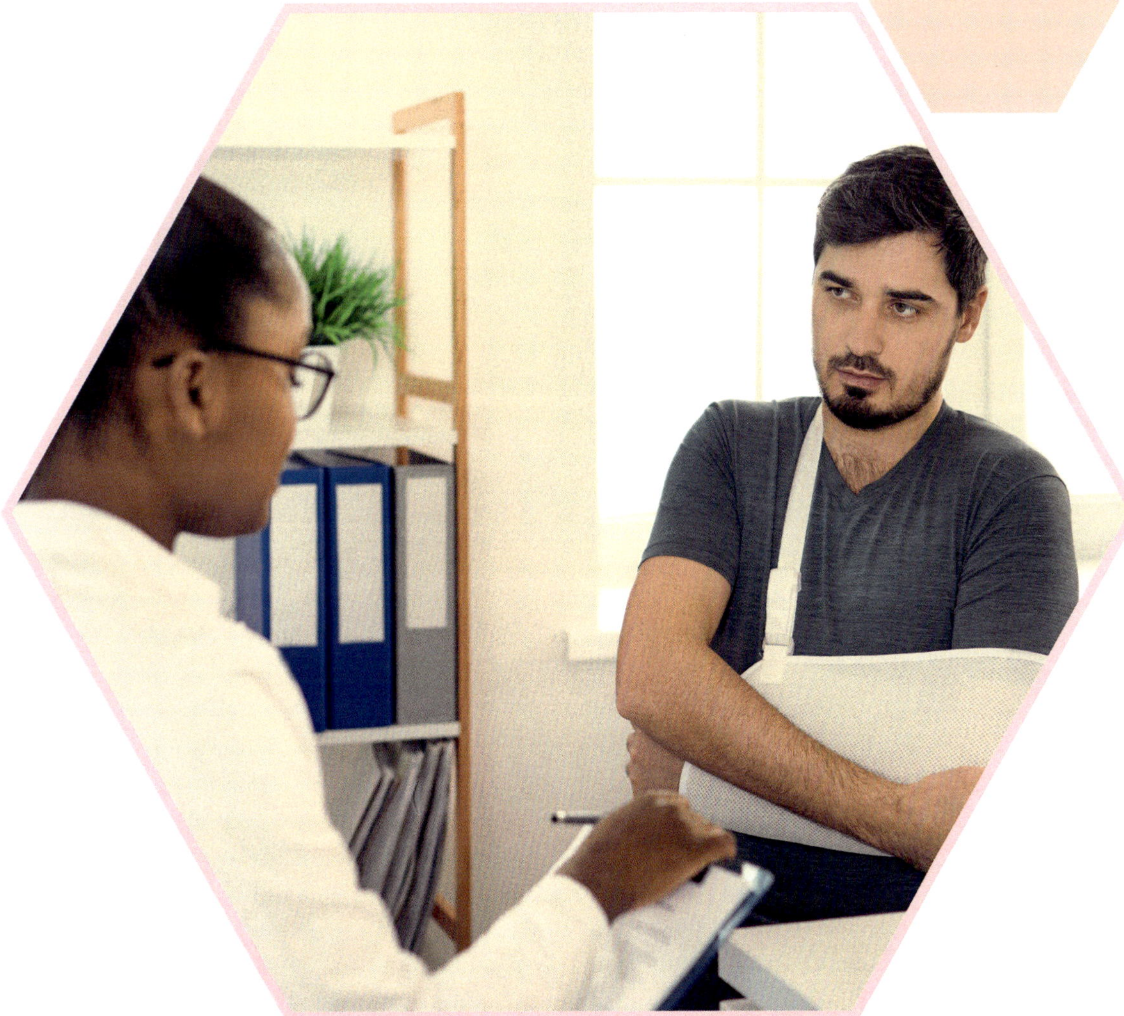

During Tommy John surgery, a surgeon will replace your UCL with a new tendon. Surgeons will remove the injured tendon, drill holes into your bone, and **anchor** a new tendon in place.

Whether surgery or RICE is recommended, it is important that you follow every instruction from your doctor. Each step of the treatment process is important and is designed to help you recover. The doctors and surgeons want to see you return to sports quickly, and following the treatment plan is the fastest way there.

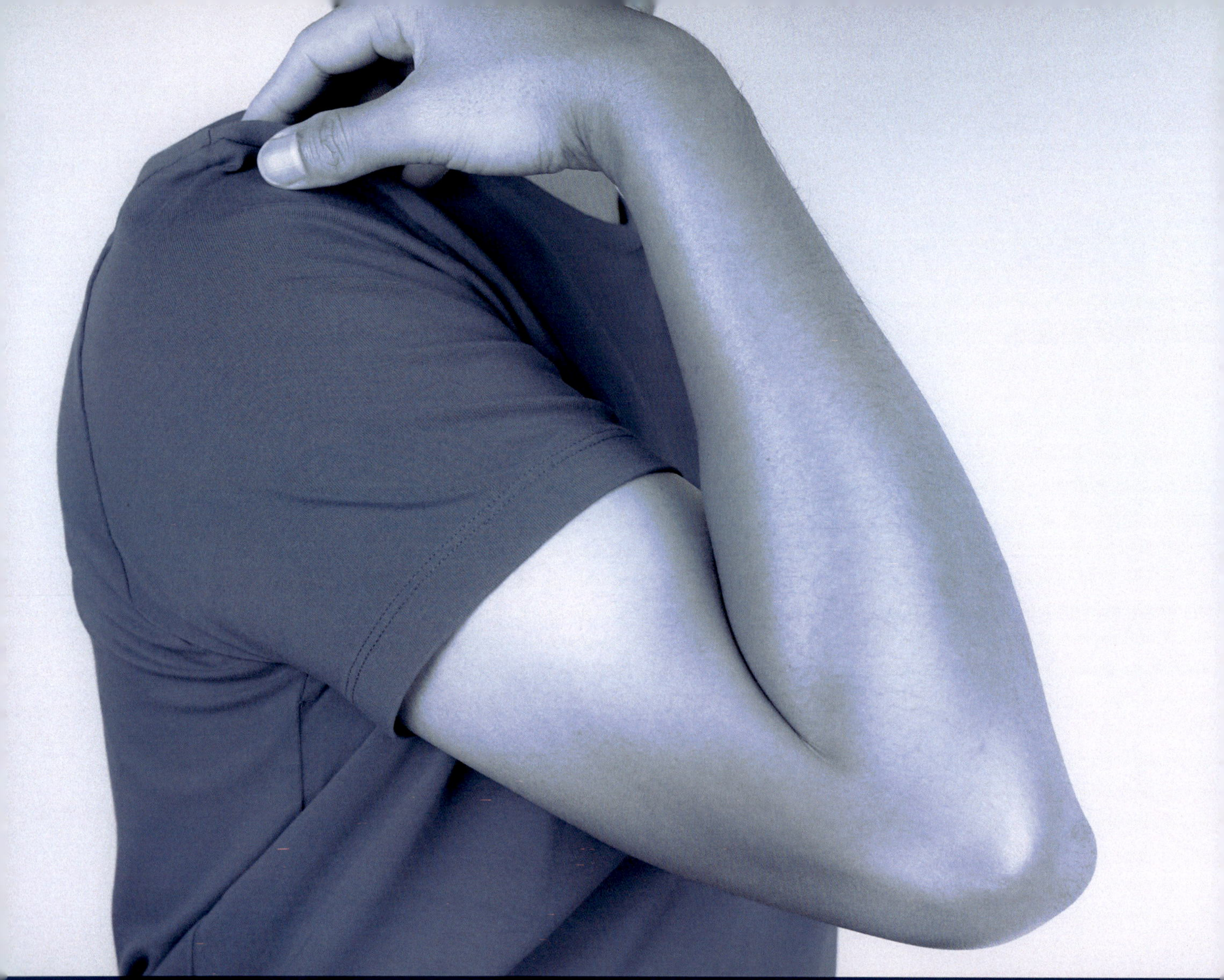

Chapter 7: Recovery

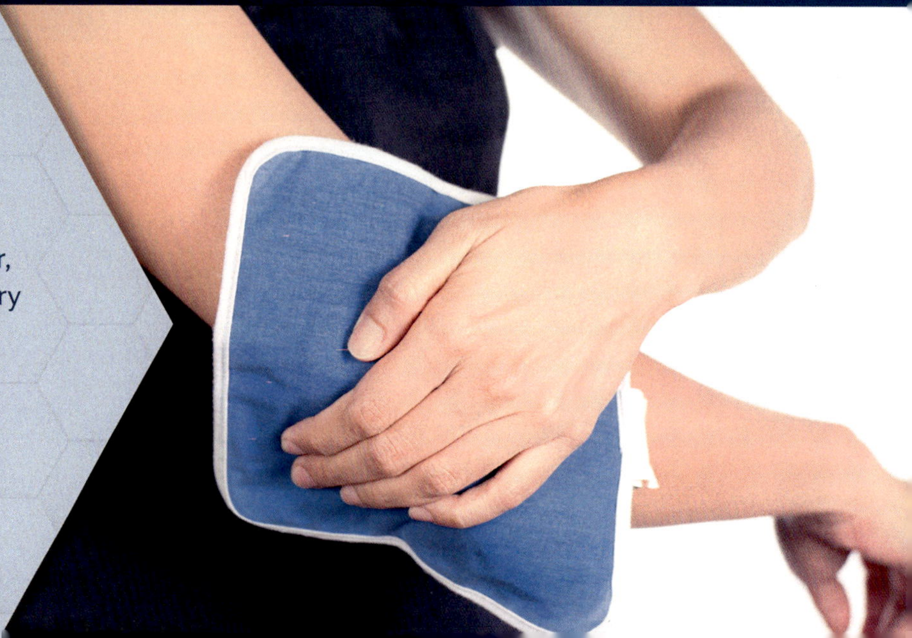

If you have a mild, Grade 1 injury, then you may recover using RICE in as little as 6 to 9 weeks. However, recovering from a more severe injury will take longer.

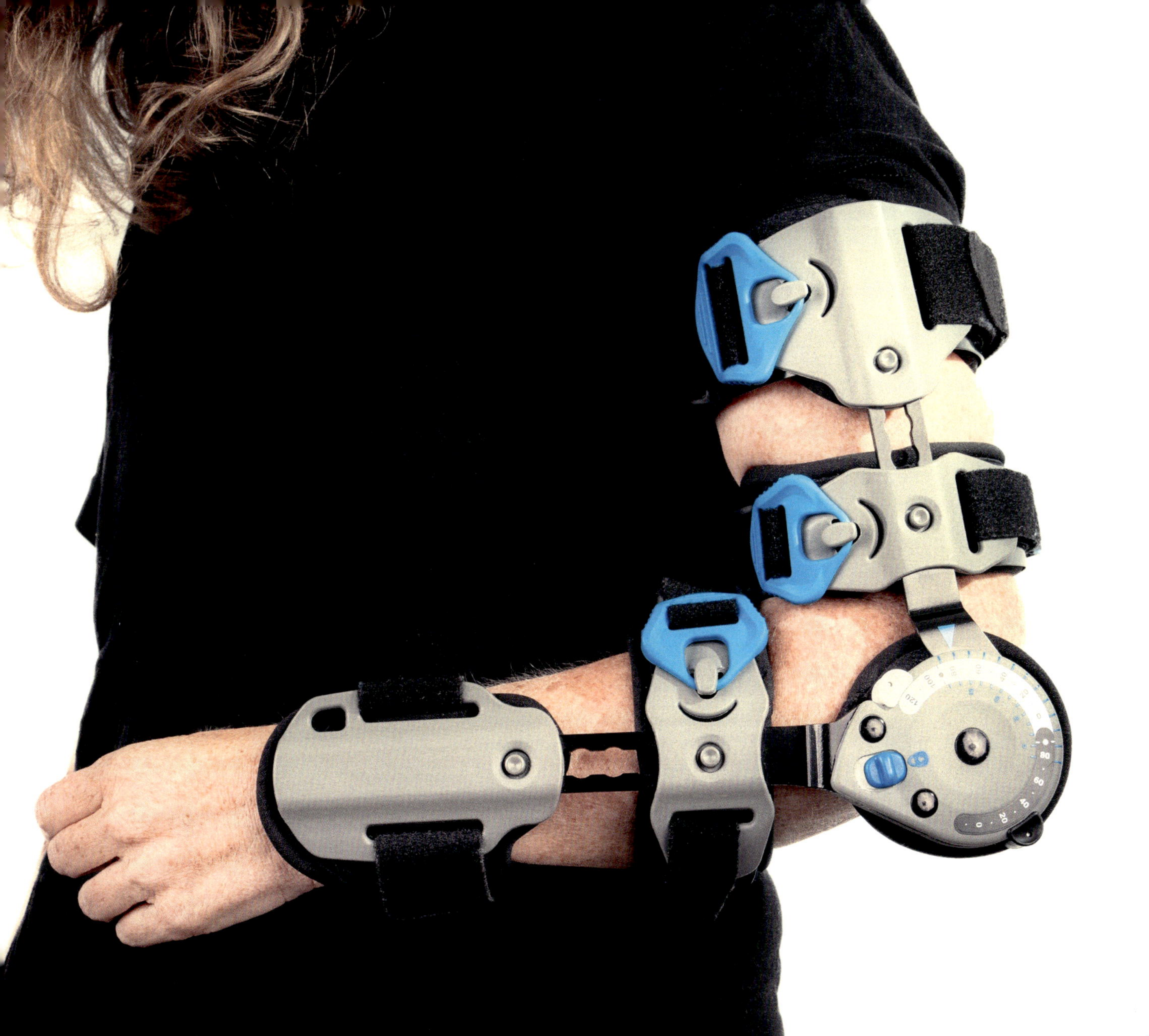

Recovering from a Tommy John surgery has several stages. Immediately after surgery, your arm will be in a brace. The brace is to support your arm and reduce swelling. A few weeks after surgery, you may be given a moveable brace or a sling. This means that your injury has healed enough that you can start moving your elbow again. You might be out of a brace completely in as little as a month after the surgery.

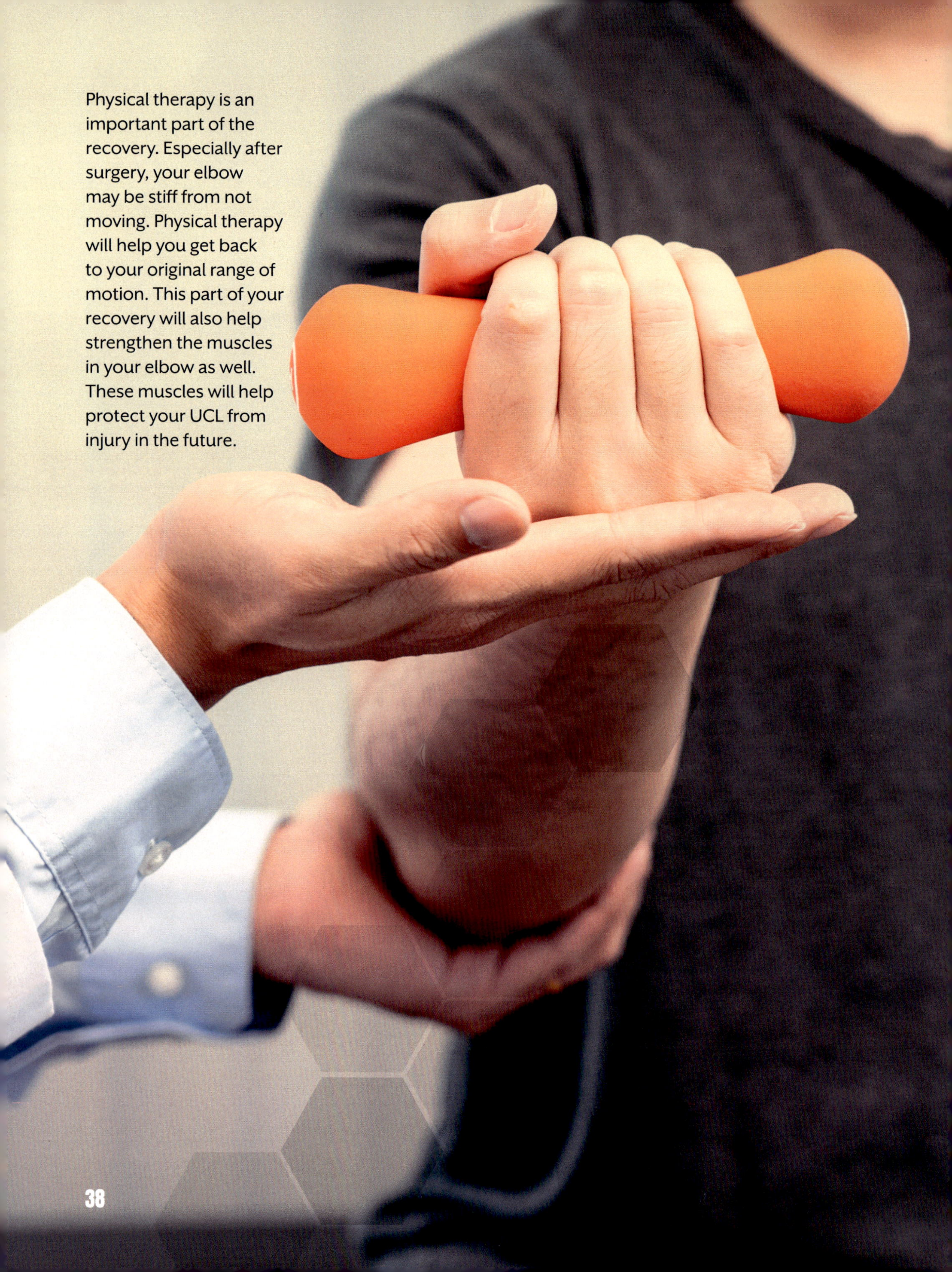

Physical therapy is an important part of the recovery. Especially after surgery, your elbow may be stiff from not moving. Physical therapy will help you get back to your original range of motion. This part of your recovery will also help strengthen the muscles in your elbow as well. These muscles will help protect your UCL from injury in the future.

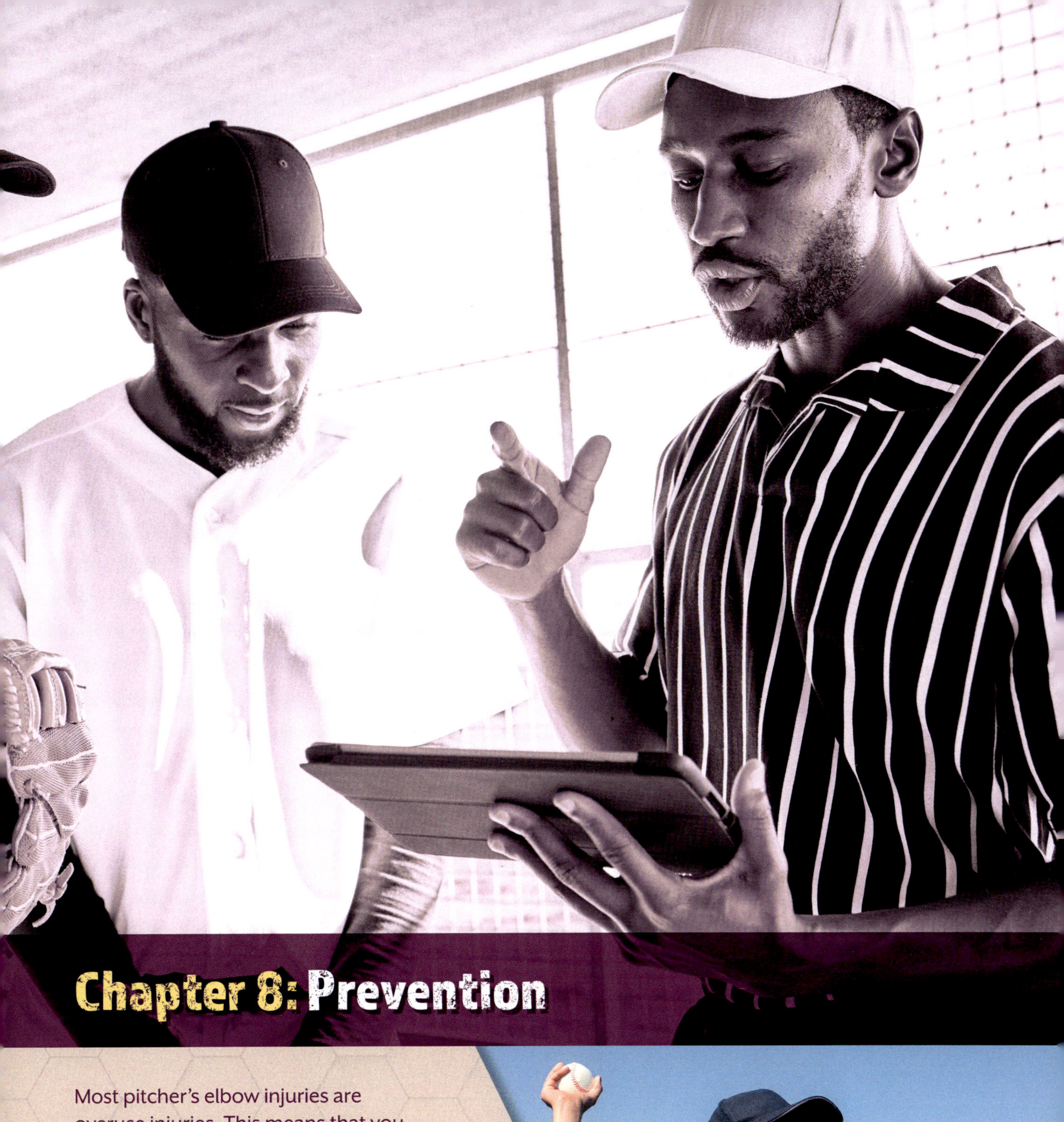

Chapter 8: Prevention

Most pitcher's elbow injuries are overuse injuries. This means that you have time to prevent the injury from occurring or from getting worse. If you play in a sport with a lot of throwing, especially if you're a baseball pitcher, talk with your coach about some of these ways of preventing pitcher's elbow injuries.

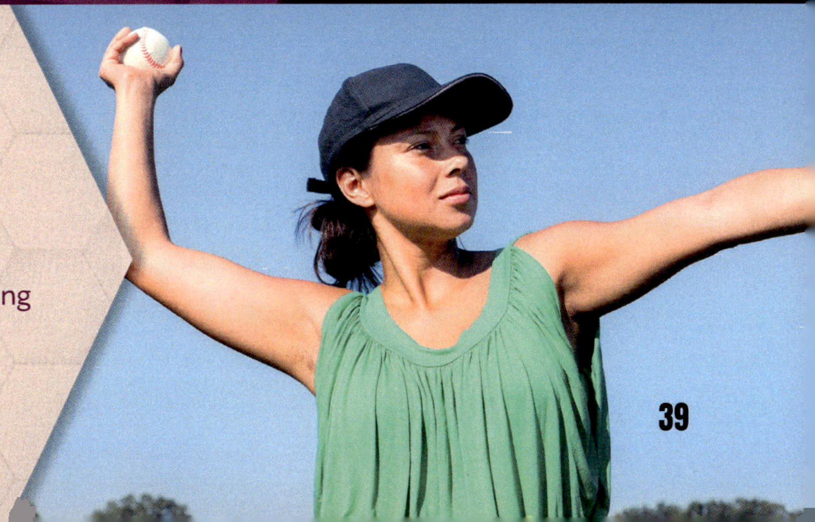

The most important factor in preventing pitcher's elbow is rest. Pain in your elbow is never a good sign, and it means that you should take a break before you become even more seriously injured. Rotating to play at other positions may help decrease your pain. Keeping count of the number of pitches you've thrown and stopping after a certain number is another way of helping you to rest.

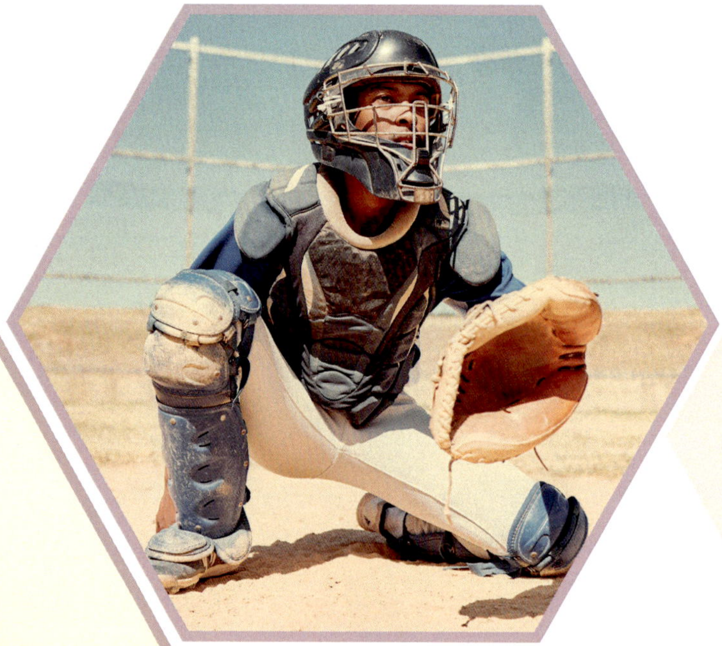

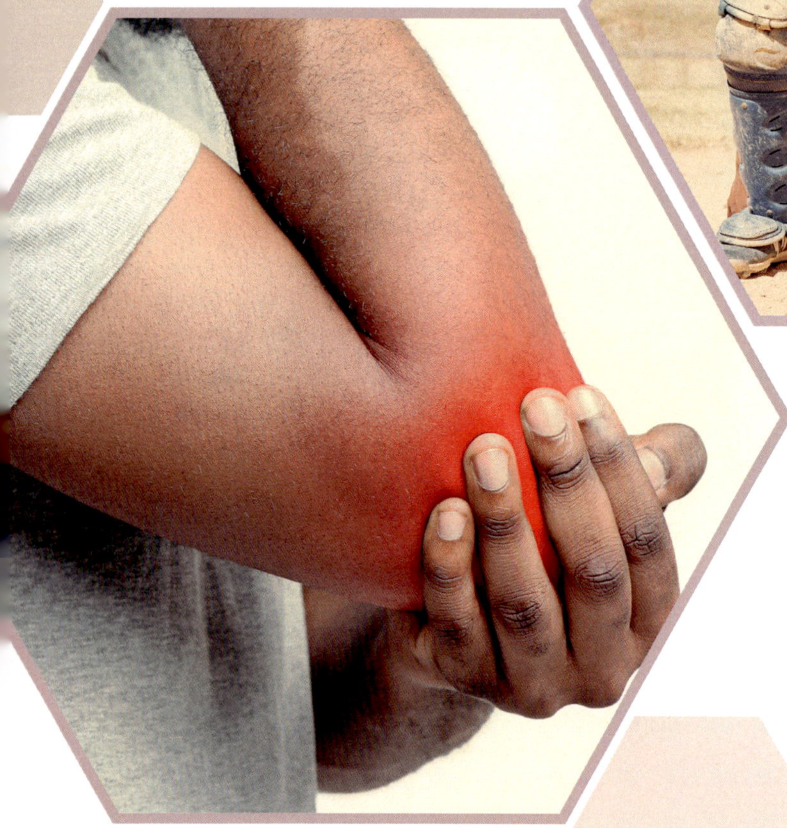

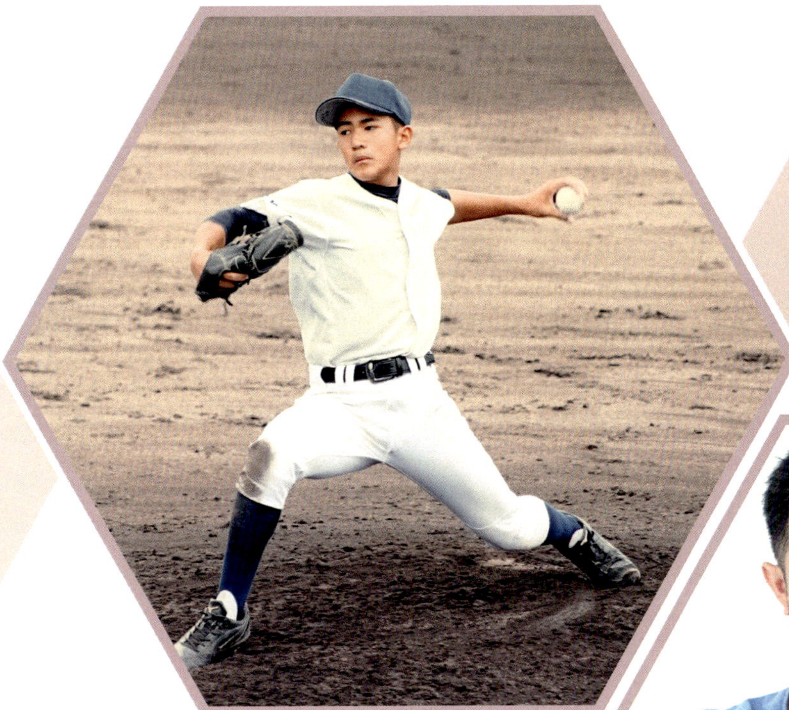

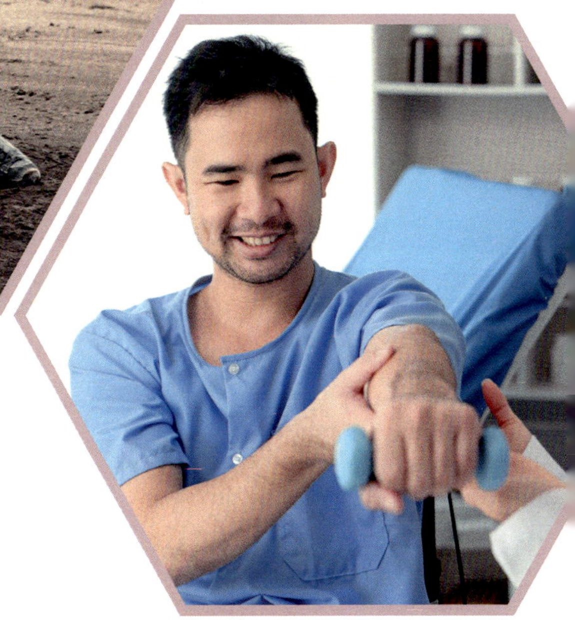

Physical therapy and coaching can help you strengthen the muscles around your elbow. These muscles can protect the UCL during throwing. Using good throwing form may also decrease the stress on your UCL and help prevent injury.

Be sure to stretch and warm up gradually before play. Start with slow throws and pitches. Increase your speed gradually. Remember that pain is a sign that something is wrong. Pushing past pain will make this overuse injury worse. Only throw and pitch as fast as you can without any pain.

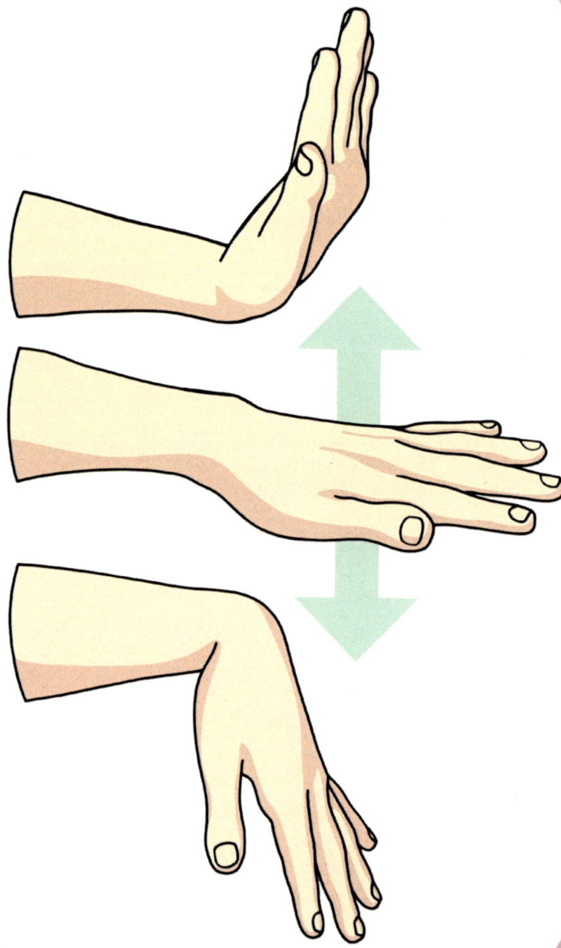

One exercise a physical therapist may suggest is a wrist curl.

1.) *Place your lower arm flat on a table with your wrist hanging off the edge.*

2.) *Slowly raise your wrist*

3.) *Slowly lower it all the way back down*

Pitcher's elbow is a common injury in throwing sports, especially in baseball. There are effective treatments, including Tommy John surgery, if you get hurt. By warming up slowly, strengthening the muscles around your elbow, and throwing with good form, you can help prevent this injury.

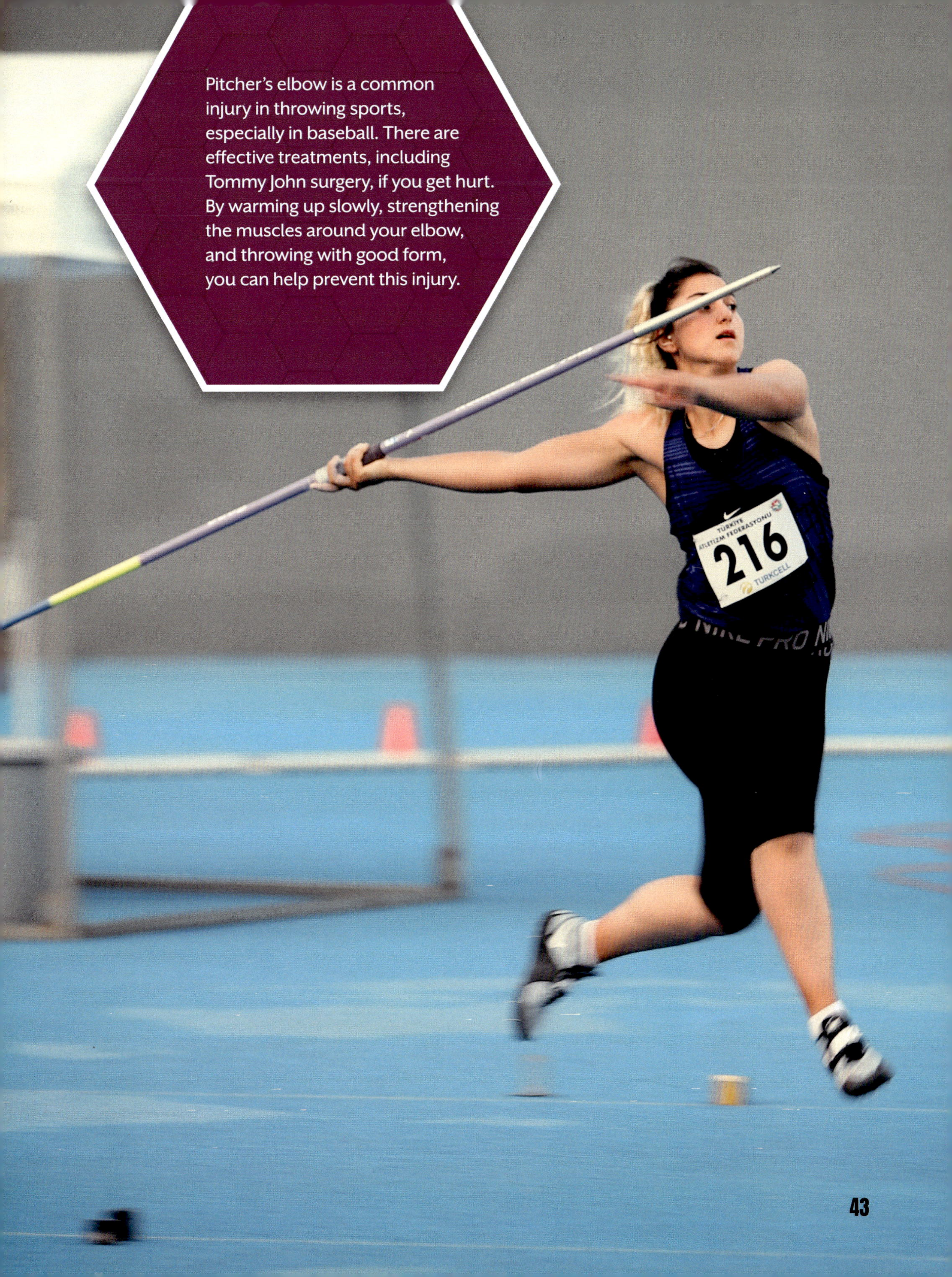

Glossary

anatomy (un-NAT-uh-mee): The study of the parts of the human body

anchor (ANG-ker): A device for holding something in place

bone (bohn): A hard material in the human body that provides structure

compress (kuhm-PRES): To press together or squeeze

dynamic (dhay-NAM-ik): In motion

extend (ik-STEND): To make the full length

flex (fleks): To bend

humerus (HYOO-mer-uhs): The long bone in the upper arm

joint (joint): Where two or more bones meet

ligament (LIG-uh-muhnts): Soft structures which connect bones with other bones

magnetic resonance imaging (mag-NET-ik REZ-uh-nuhns IM-uh-jing): A machine that uses magnets to take images of the soft parts inside the human body, commonly known as MRI

mobile joint (MOH-buhl joints): A joint whose purpose is to move

pronation (pro-NEY-shuhn): Counterclockwise rotation of your arm so that your palm points downward

radius (REY-dee-uhs): The long bone of the lower arm on the thumb side

range of motion (reynj uhv MOH-shun): How far a joint is able to move

supination (soo-puh-NEY-shuhn): Clockwise rotation of your arm so that your palm points upward

ulna (UHL-nuh): The long bone of the lower arm on the little finger (or pinkie) side

ultrasound (UHL-truh-sound): High frequency sound waves that are used to see inside the human body

valgus (VAL-guhs): To move away

valgus stress test (VAL-guhs stres test): When a doctor moves the lower arm away from the upper arm to determine if there is a UCL injury

X-ray (EKS-rey): Electromagnetic radiation with a shorter wavelength than light that can show images of hard tissue like bone

Index

Comprehension Questions

1. What is another name for a pitcher's elbow injury?
   a. Timmy Jimbo
   b. Thayer Justin
   c. Tommy John
2. True or false: Pitcher's elbow injuries are common sports injuries.
3. An over-use injury
   a. Happens gradually over time
   b. Usually occurs with a loud "pop!"
   c. Only happens during long games
4. True or false: Surgery is usually needed for severe pitcher's elbow injuries
5. True or false: Valgus is a medical term that means to swing
6. RICE stands for
   a. Running, Ice skating, Climbing, and Equestrian.
   b. Red, Inflamed, Contusion, and Enlarged.
   c. Rest, Ice, Compression, and Elevation.
7. One way to prevent pitcher's elbow injuries is to
   a. Limit throwing time
   b. Drink water with ice in it
   c. Exercise in shorts
8. True or false: an athlete who plays any sport with throwing can get pitcher's elbow

1. c 2. true 3. a 4. true 5. false 6. c 7. a 8. true

About the Author

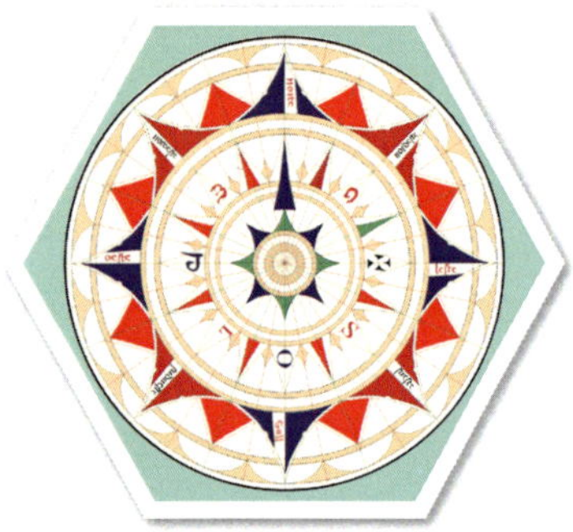

India James writes about science, technology, and math for young readers. She loves when science comes together with sports. India lives in Ohio with her family.

Author: India James
Editor: Ellen Rodger
Design: Jen Bowers

IMAGE CREDITS

Shutterstock: Cover and title page ©2022 Cinefootage Visuals (p.4, p.11, p.34), ©2023 PeopleImages.com-Yuri A (p.6), ©2023 PeopleImages.com-Yuri A (p.20), ©2020 TheCorgi (p.38); p.4 ©2018 JoeSAPhotos; p.5 ©2023 BigBlueStudio, © 2024 Conor P. Fitzgerald; p.6 ©2018 EvrenKalinbacak; p.7 ©2018 dotshock, ©2023 LightField Studios; p.8 ©2019 Orla; p.9 ©2015 Sebastian Kaulitzki; p.10 ©2022 PeopleImages.com-Yuri A, ©2024 Toru Kimura; p.11 ©2020 New Africa; p.12 ©2023 BigBlueStudio; p.13 ©Alila Medical Media; p.14 ©2016 Sebastian Kaulitzki, ©2019 Regreto; p.15 ©2018 Andrew Cline; p.16 ©2023 PeopleImages.com-Yuri A; p.17 ©2024 Mr.Teerapong Kunkaeo, ©2013 Nomad_Soul; p.18 © 2022 Master1305; p.19 ©2023 Sebastian Kaulitzki, ©2020 Dean Drobot; p.20 ©2023 ViDI Studio; p.21 ©Pepermpron (p.31); p.22 ©2022 PeopleImages.com-Yuri A, ©2021 DC Studio; p.23 ©2021 Tom Wang, ©2021 wutzkohphoto; p.24 ©2023 djile; p.25 ©2024 New Africa; p.26 ©2023 Wasan Tita; p.27 ©2021 fizkes, ©2017 Derya Cakirsoy; p.28 ©2024 Svitlana Hulko; p.29 ©2017 Africa Studio; p.30 ©2023 YAKOBCHUK VIACHESLAV, ©2016 kaling2100; p.31 ©2022 Studio Romantic; p.32 ©2020 Wira SHK, ©2024 Krakenimages.com, ©2019 New Africa; p.33 ©2019 mdbildes, © 2015 Peter Titmuss; p.34 ©2015 Chaikom; p.35 ©2021 Studio Romantic; p.36 ©2024 Aria Armoko, ©2016 Chutima Chaochaiya; p.37 ©2023 sophiecat; p.39 ©2023 PeopleImages.com-Yuri A, ©2017 Ben Schonewille; p.40 ©2020 Prostock-studio, ©2022 PeopleImages.com-Yuri A; p.41 ©2024 Primo Passo, ©2024 CrizzyStudio; p.42 ©Hakan Kutlu; p.43 ©2021 EvrenKalinbacak; p.48 About the Author image ©Alvesgaspar

Crabtree Publishing

crabtreebooks.com 800-387-7650

In Canada: We acknowledge the financial support of the Government of Canada through the Canada Book Fund for our publishing activities.

Hardcover 978-1-0398-8081-8
Paperback 978-1-0398-8442-7
Ebook (pdf) 978-1-0398-8201-0
Epub 978-1-0398-8321-5

Published in Canada
Crabtree Publishing
616 Welland Avenue
St. Catharines, Ontario
L2M 5V6

Published in the United States
Crabtree Publishing
347 Fifth Avenue
Suite 1402-145
New York, New York, 10016

Library and Archives Canada Cataloguing in Publication
Available at Library and Archives Canada

Library of Congress Cataloging-in-Publication Data
Available at the Library of Congress

Printed in the USA/CP2025